Evidence-Based Procedures in Facial Plastic Surgery

Editors

LISA E. ISHII
TRAVIS T. TOLLEFSON

FACIAL PLASTIC SURGERY CLINICS OF NORTH AMERICA

www.facialplastic.theclinics.com

Consulting Editor
J. REGAN THOMAS

August 2015 • Volume 23 • Number 3

ELSEVIER

1600 John F. Kennedy Boulevard • Suite 1800 • Philadelphia, Pennsylvania, 19103-2899

http://www.theclinics.com

FACIAL PLASTIC SURGERY CLINICS OF NORTH AMERICA Volume 23, Number 3
August 2015 ISSN 1064-7406, ISBN-13: 978-0-323-39332-4

Editor: Joanne Husovski
Developmental Editor: Susan Showalter

Facial Plastic Surgery Clinics of North America (ISSN 1064-7406) is published quarterly by Elsevier Inc., 360 Park Avenue South, New York, NY 10010-1710. Months of issue are February, May, August, and November. Business and Editorial Offices: 1600 John F. Kennedy Blvd., Suite 1800, Philadelphia, PA 19103-2899. Periodicals postage paid at New York, NY, and additional mailing offices. Subscription prices are $390.00 per year (US individuals), $525.00 per year (US institutions), $445.00 per year (Canadian individuals), $653.00 per year (Canadian institutions), $535.00 per year (foreign individuals), $653.00 per year (foreign institutions), $185.00 per year (US students), and $255.00 per year (foreign students). Foreign air speed delivery is included in all *Clinics* subscription prices. All prices are subject to change without notice. POSTMASTER: Send address changes to *Facial Plastic Surgery Clinics*, Elsevier Health Sciences Division, Subscription Customer Service, 3251 Riverport Lane, Maryland Heights, MO 63043. **Customer service: 1-800-654-2452 (US and Canada); 1-314-447-8871 (outside US and Canada); Fax: 314-447-8029; E-mail: journalscustomerservice-usa@elsevier.com (for print support); journalsonline support-usa@elsevier.com (for online support).**

Reprints. For copies of 100 or more of articles in this publication, please contact the Commercial Reprints Department, Elsevier Inc., 360 Park Avenue South, New York, NY 10010-1710. Tel.: 212-633-3874; Fax: 212-633-3820; E-mail: reprints@elsevier.com.

Facial Plastic Surgery Clinics of North America is covered in *MEDLINE/PubMed* (*Index Medicus*).

Contributors

CONSULTING EDITOR

J. REGAN THOMAS, MD, FACS
Professor and Chairman, Department of
Otolaryngology, University of Illinois at
Chicago, Chicago, Illinois

EDITORS

LISA E. ISHII, MD, MHS
Associate Professor, Department of
Otolaryngology–Head and Neck Surgery,
Johns Hopkins School of Medicine, Baltimore,
Maryland

TRAVIS T. TOLLEFSON, MD, MPH, FACS
Associate Professor, Facial Plastic and
Reconstructive Surgery, Department of
Otolaryngology–Head and Neck Surgery,
University of California-Davis, Sacramento,
California

AUTHORS

MICHAEL J. BRENNER, MD, FACS
Associate Professor, Division of Facial Plastic
and Reconstructive Surgery, Department of
Otolaryngology–Head and Neck Surgery,
University of Michigan School of Medicine,
Ann Arbor, Michigan

STEVEN B. CANNADY, MD
Department of Otolaryngology–Head and Neck
Surgery, University of Pennsylvania,
Philadelphia, Pennsylvania

J. JARED CHRISTOPHEL, MD, MPH
Department of Otolaryngology–Head and Neck
Surgery, University of Virginia Health System,
Charlottesville, Virginia

AMELIA CLARK, MD
Resident in Otolaryngology, Head and Neck
Surgery, Stanford University, Palo Alto,
California

TIMOTHY D. DOERR, MD, FACS
Associate Professor, Director of Facial Plastic
Surgery, Department of Otolaryngology–Head
and Neck Surgery, University of Rochester
School of Medicine and Dentistry, Rochester,
New York

TESSA A. HADLOCK, MD
Director, Division of Facial Plastic and
Reconstructive Surgery, Department of
Otolaryngology; Director, Facial Nerve
Center, Massachusetts Eye and Ear Infirmary,
Harvard Medical School, Boston,
Massachusetts

BASIL HASSOUNEH, MD
Lecturer, Department of Otolaryngology–
Head and Neck Surgery, University of
Toronto; Eye Face Institute, Toronto,
Ontario, Canada

JILL L. HESSLER, MD
Medical Director of Hessler Plastic
Surgery, Adjunct Clinical Assistant
Professor of Otolaryngology, Head and
Neck Surgery, Stanford University,
Palo Alto, California

DAVID HYMAN, MD
Section of Facial Plastic Surgery, Division of
Otolaryngology, Department of Surgery,
University of Wisconsin, Madison,
Wisconsin

NATE JOWETT, MD
Clinical Fellow, Division of Facial Plastic and Reconstructive Surgery, Department of Otolaryngology, Facial Nerve Center, Massachusetts Eye and Ear Infirmary, Harvard Medical School, Boston, Massachusetts

ROBERT G. KELLER, MD
Resident, Department of Otolaryngology–Head and Neck Surgery, Medical University of South Carolina, Charleston, South Carolina

ERIC LAMARRE, MD
Department of Otolaryngology–Head and Neck Surgery, Cleveland Clinic Foundation, Cleveland, Ohio

MATTHEW K. LEE, MD
Clinical Instructor, Division of Facial Plastic and Reconstructive Surgery, Stanford University School of Medicine, Stanford, California

C. CARRIE LIU, MD
Division of Otolaryngology–Head and Neck Surgery, Department of Surgery, Foothills Medical Centre, University of Calgary, Calgary, Alberta, Canada

BENJAMIN C. MARCUS, MD
Section of Facial Plastic Surgery, Division of Otolaryngology, Department of Surgery, University of Wisconsin, Madison, Wisconsin

SAM P. MOST, MD
Chief, Division of Facial Plastic and Reconstructive Surgery; Professor, Department of Otolaryngology–Head and Neck Surgery, Stanford University School of Medicine, Stanford, California

KRISHNA G. PATEL, MD, PhD
Assistant Professor, Facial Plastic and Reconstructive Surgery, Department of Otolaryngology–Head and Neck Surgery, Medical University of South Carolina, Charleston, South Carolina

DAVID SHAYE, MD
Division of Facial Plastic and Reconstructive Surgery, Massachusetts Eye and Ear Infirmary, Harvard Medical School, Boston, Massachusetts

JAMES TENG, MD
Department of Otolaryngology–Head and Neck Surgery, University of Virginia Health System, Charlottesville, Virginia

TRAVIS T. TOLLEFSON, MD, MPH, FACS
Associate Professor, Facial Plastic and Reconstructive Surgery, Department of Otolaryngology–Head and Neck Surgery, University of California-Davis, Sacramento, California

MARK K. WAX, MD
Department of Otolaryngology–Head and Neck Surgery, Oregon Health and Sciences University, Portland, Oregon

Contents

> Systematic reviews and meta-analyses hold a unique position in the pyramid of evidence. They can provide transparent and rigorous summaries to answer many clinical questions in facial plastic surgery. They can also identify areas of research deficiency, create new knowledge, and support guidelines or policies. A well-conducted systematic review follows a structured process to minimize bias and ensure reproducibility. When appropriate, a meta-analysis is incorporated to provide a statistical synthesis that combines the results of individual studies. This powerful quantitative method is becoming more prevalent in facial plastic surgery. This article provides a practical framework to understand and conduct this valuable type of research.

> Aging skin is among the most common patient concerns in a facial plastic surgery practice. Ultraviolet (UV)-induced damage expedites the pace of intrinsic aging, resulting in many of the visible signs of aging, such as rough skin texture, pigmentation irregularities, fine and deep wrinkling, and inelasticity. Primary prevention of UV and environmental damage with proper skin care and the use of sunscreen are critical. There is great interest in topically applied products to reverse or delay the visible signs of photoaging. We discuss the most common topically applied agents for photoaging, reviewing their mechanisms and supporting evidence.

> In the setting of rapidly changing technology tone must make a decision on whether he or she places a premium on being an "early adopter" of technology or delay purchasing decisions until there is adequate proof that a particular technology is useful. Laser devices are a significant capital expenditure, and therefore members of the second group who base their purchasing decisions on evidence-based medicine may be able to avoid deploying capitol into a purchase that becomes obsolete as quickly as it appeared.

> Evidence-based medicine has become increasingly prominent in the climate of modern day healthcare. The practice of evidence-based medicine involves the integration of the best available evidence with clinical experience and expertise to help guide clinical decision-making. The essential tenets of evidence-based medicine can be applied to both functional and aesthetic rhinoplasty. Current outcome

measures in functional and aesthetic rhinoplasty, including objective, subjective, and clinician-reported measures, is summarized and the current data is reviewed.

This article provides an overview of the current state of the art of facial reanimation using the best available evidence. Medical, surgical, and physical therapy options in acute and long-standing facial palsy are discussed.

With demands for an evidence-based approach to patient care, the management of facial fractures will come under increasing scrutiny because there is an overall deficiency in higher level clinical evidence. This article reviews the management of facial fractures, focusing on an evidence-based approach. It focuses on select areas of facial trauma in which there is controversy and presents randomized studies and meta-analysis to help define best practice. The article notes the many areas where the evidenced-based literature is weak and looks at the future of evidence-based facial trauma care.

Microvascular free tissue transfer is the best modality of replacing composite tissue defects with composite vascularized tissue. Wound healing, functional reconstruction, rehabilitation, and cosmesis are best accomplished when the tissue defect is replaced by free tissue. The reconstructive tissue can be tailored to the defect and is harvested from outside the often radiated pretreated reconstructive field. Evidence to support the use of free tissue transfer in head and neck defects is not of the highest level. This article reviews the postoperative monitoring of free tissue transfer, lateral mandibular reconstruction (fibula vs radial forearm), and functional outcomes with free tissue transfers.

The current article reviews the pertinent literature on the management of cleft lip and palate. We review the commonly used surgical techniques for repair, adjunctive options for treatment, clinical outcomes, complications, and concerns to consider. Throughout the discussion, we state the level of evidence where applicable and identify areas for future study.

Over the past decade, the treatment of infantile hemangiomas has undergone dramatic breakthroughs. This review critically evaluates the latest literature that supports the myriad treatment options for infantile hemangiomas. It chronicles the fading role of steroid therapy and evolution of propranolol use as the major treatment modality. Although propranolol is helping this disease become more of a medical disease and less of a surgical dilemma, the report also reveals a continued search to find nonsystemic treatment options. In summary, this is an evidence-based medicine review for the treatment of infantile hemangiomas.

The practice of evidence-based medicine combines physician experience, knowledge of current literature, and patient preferences. Different grading systems are used to evaluate current levels of evidence and recommendations. A variety of common instruments are used to measure outcomes in facial plastic surgery. These instruments are used for expert data collection, including assessment of pathology and response to treatment, or for patient-reported outcome measures, including quality of life, disability, and daily function. Integration of data collection requires storage and protection of health information. We provide an outline to what is involved in understanding evidence-based medicine and incorporating it into daily practice.

FACIAL PLASTIC SURGERY CLINICS OF NORTH AMERICA

THE CLINICS ARE AVAILABLE ONLINE!
Access your subscription at:
www.theclinics.com

Preface

Evidence-Based Procedures in Facial Plastic and Reconstructive Surgery

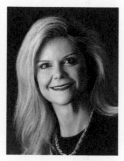
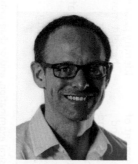

Lisa E. Ishii, MD, MHS   Travis T. Tollefson, MD, MPH, FACS

Editors

While our specialty has experienced exciting successes, advances, and important contributions to patient care, evidenced by a cadre of satisfied patients and providers, we have the opportunity to take these results to the next level. Until recently, the effectiveness of facial plastic and reconstructive interventions has been evaluated primarily by subjective opinion and retrospective chart reviews. Furthermore, many physicians base patient care decisions on historical perspectives and personal experience.

Over the last several years, the practice of medicine shifted toward an evidence-based medicine (EBM) approach that "de-emphasizes intuition, unsystematic clinical experience, and pathophysiologic rationale as sufficient grounds for clinical decision making and stresses the examination of evidence from clinical research."[1] Physicians have been moving away from reliance primarily on expert opinion to instead supplement their practice and clinical expertise with the other two major pillars in EBM, namely, best research evidence and patient values.[2] Sackett and colleagues[3] suggest that this is a "conscience, explicit, and judicious use of the current best evidence in making decisions about the care of individual patients."

The Oxford Center for Evidence-based Medicine introduced the "Level of Evidence" categorization to evaluate clinical evidence.[4] Within this model of categorization, the highest category of evidence,

level I, includes the properly powered and well-conducted randomized control trials or systematic reviews/meta-analysis of those randomized control trials. Level II evidence includes well-designed control trials that exist without randomization, or prospective comparative cohort trials. Level III evidence includes case control studies, retrospective cohort studies, and cross-sectional studies. Level IV evidence includes those case series that provide descriptive information about the set of patient characteristics. Level V evidence includes case reports and expert opinions and has previously been the mainstay of evaluation in Facial Plastic and Reconstructive Surgery.

Multifactorial occurrences supported the paradigm shift toward more evidence-based analysis of surgical outcomes. First, the development of technologically advanced treatments requires comparative effectiveness to determine cost-effectiveness of these over the traditional management. Next, public and private payers link reimbursement to patient outcomes and satisfaction. Last, unacceptable variation in process and outcome measures and cost exists nationally for common procedures. This combination of factors, among others, contributes to the proliferation of hypothesis testing with research question development using PICOTS (**Table 1**).

The development of high-quality outcomes research is dependent on accurate and reproducible

Facial Plast Surg Clin N Am 23 (2015) ix–xii
http://dx.doi.org/10.1016/j.fsc.2015.06.001
1064-7406/15/$ – see front matter © 2015 Published by Elsevier Inc.

Table 1
PICOTS format as a framework for developing research questions

Component	Comment	Diagnosis Question Example[a]	Treatment/Harm Question Example[b]	Prognosis Question Example[c]
Population	Patient, population, or problem to which the question applies	Adults with acute upper respiratory infection	Adults with acute bacterial sinusitis	Adults with acute bacterial sinusitis
Intervention	Service, planned action, prognostic factor, or cause of interest	History, physical examination, or diagnostic test	Antibiotic therapy for 7 to 10 days	Prognostic factors, including age, illness severity, comorbid conditions (eg, allergic rhinitis)
Comparator (optional)	When applicable, an alternative intervention or comparison	None	Placebo or no therapy	None
Outcome(s)	Measurements to determine the impact of the intervention and comparator	Distinguish bacterial vs viral sinusitis	Clinical improvement of presenting signs and symptoms; harms and adverse events	Identify patients who are likely to benefit most from antibiotic therapy
Time frame (optional)	Timing or time frame of interest	Within the first 3 weeks of illness	During and after treatment	During and after treatment
Setting (optional)	Clinical care or other setting of interest	Any setting	Any setting	Any setting

[a] The PICOTS question would be the following: "For adults with acute upper respiratory infection, how can history, physical examination, and/or diagnostic tests be used to distinguish bacterial from viral infection within the first 3 weeks of illness?"
[b] The PICOTS question would be the following: "For adults with acute bacterial sinusitis, what is the impact of antibiotic therapy for 7 to 10 days vs placebo or no therapy on clinical improvement (of presenting signs and symptoms) and on adverse events during and after treatment?"
[c] The PICOTS question would be the following: "For adults with acute bacterial sinusitis, what prognostic factors (eg, age, illness, severity, comorbid conditions) can be used to identify patients most likely to benefit from antibiotic therapy during and after treatment?"
From Rosenfeld RM, Shiffman RN, Robertson P. Clinical Practice Guideline Development Manual, Third Edition: a quality-driven approach for translating evidence into action. Otolaryngol Head Neck Surg 2013;148(1 Suppl):S1–55; with permission.

measurement tools. If the outcomes of reconstructive or esthetic facial surgery are to be compared between surgeons, centers, or health care systems, we need to agree on reliable, standardized data collection processes. These data standards are arduous, but necessary for comparative effectiveness research. For example, researchers are testing research questions in new technologies to determine the clinical relevance and applicability, which include the following: intraoperative imaging for craniomaxillofacial trauma,[5] photography software for facial reanimation outcomes,[6] and video nasopharyngoscopy for cleft palate-related speech surgeries. Patient-oriented outcomes evaluating health-related quality of life and perception of outcomes are increasingly important.[7–9]

The objective of this issue of *Facial Plastic Surgery Clinics of North America* is to describe the state-of-the-science of EBM in the field of Facial Plastic and Reconstructive Surgery. This special issue is devoted to contributions from forward thinkers in EBM approaches. The general overview of systematic reviews and meta-analysis is provided first to introduce the framework by which previous research can be gathered and synthesized to obtain the best available evidence. Dr Brennan distilled this complex topic into an easy-to-understand primer for even the beginner in EBM. One of the most difficult areas to ascertain comparative effectiveness is within the use of skin care products in cosmetic facial plastic surgery clinics. Drs Hessler and Clark have provided a review of the best evidence for the effectiveness of the most commonly recommended cosmetic skin treatment programs. Dr Hyman and Marcus compiled a comparative article evaluating the pros and cons of different laser options for the treatments ranging from treating pigmentation abnormalities, aging face, or congenital vascular malformations. Drs Lee and Most present a succinct comparison of rhinoplasty outcomes and analysis. Improved data collection in rhinoplasty is advocated to enable comparative outcomes assessment.

Reconstructive surgical procedures for facial reanimation are reviewed by Drs Jowett and Hadlock, in which the quality-of-life outcomes, standardized photograph analysis, and other outcome parameters are described as they have been developed at the Massachusetts Eye and Ear Infirmary. Facial trauma and modern management techniques are reviewed as comparative craniomaxillofacial fixation and reduction techniques have emerged over the last several decades. Dr Doerr has summarized some of the controversial topics and compared the evidence to support each side. Drs Cannady, Lamarre,

and Wax have evaluated the evidence for both the current state of functional outcomes and the management protocols for microvascular free tissue transfer in craniomaxillofacial surgical reconstruction, including intraoperative monitoring. Drs Shaye, Liu, and Tollefson reviewed the most recent evidence supporting management choices, including timing and procedure choices for children with cleft lip and palate. Drs Keller and Patel have created a careful review of the modern management philosophies for facial vascular anomalies, which include the true breakthrough of nonsurgical treatment with propranolol becoming more of the mainstay primary treatment.

Last, Drs Teng and Christophel provide the early practice focus section as a primer for EBM practice in Facial Plastic Surgery. They summarized what is meant by an evidence-based practice. This format is to allow any reader to grasp the concept of developing research questions with reproducible collection of outcomes. This how-to manual gives concrete examples of the manner with which a newly practicing or seasoned surgeon might collect data to allow comparisons, develop research questions, evaluate the current evidence, and develop evidence-based practice decisions.

EVIDENCE-BASED MEDICINE AND OPTIMIZING CARE VALUE

In all disciplines of medicine, we are beginning to realize the full potential of EBM to improve the value of patient care. As data from high levels of evidence (LOE) studies have proliferated, those data have been used to create Clinical Practice Guidelines (CPGs). CPGs are instruments that make patient management recommendations for providers based on aggregated high-level evidence, typically from systematic reviews and randomized controlled trials. The Institute of Medicine, in its brief report in 2011, noted that trustworthy CPGs should contain eight specific elements and be easily implemented by physicians and other care providers to optimize patient care.[10]

CPGs, in addition to making patient care recommendations, serve as a platform for the development of performance measures. These performance measures can in turn be used for quality reporting and demonstrating the value of our care to all stakeholders, namely, patients, providers, and payers alike (**Fig. 1**). For example, the American Academy of Otolaryngology–Head and Neck Surgery developed a sinusitis performance measure group based on the recommendations in the sinusitis CPG. The sinusitis CPG in turn was developed through the critical appraisal and

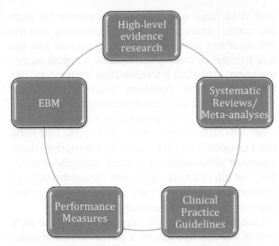

Fig. 1. Continuous cycle connecting high-level research and EBM.

aggregation of evidence from systematic reviews.[11] It was used to develop a performance measure group that providers can use for PQRS (patient quality reporting system) reporting.

Thus, as we design research using rigorous methodology and implement findings from high-level research in our practice, we ultimately see the impact of our evidence translated to our patients and improving value in measurable ways. These advances enable us to objectively demonstrate the quality of the care we provide in a manner previously not possible. In our own specialty, Facial Plastic and Reconstructive Surgery, we are on the cusp of making treatment recommendations to our patients based on high-level evidence in a manner that optimizes care for our patients. Furthermore, this enables us to objectively demonstrate the value of our care to patients and payers alike. We can all imagine a time when high-level studies distinguish which type of intervention is best for specific disease conditions, and we can use that information to educate our patients. Furthermore, this will obviate debating treatments with payers who question them.

We hope you enjoy this issue of *Facial Plastic Surgery Clinics of North America*.

Lisa E. Ishii, MD, MHS
Department of Otolaryngology–
Head & Neck Surgery
Johns Hopkins School of Medicine
Baltimore, MD 21287, USA

Travis T. Tollefson, MD, MPH, FACS
Facial Plastic and Reconstructive Surgery
Department of Otolaryngology–
Head and Neck Surgery
University of California-Davis
Sacramento, CA 95817, USA

E-mail addresses:
Learnes2@jhmi.edu (L.E. Ishii)
tttollefson@ucdavis.edu (T.T. Tollefson)

REFERENCES

1. Evidence-Based Medicine Working Group. Evidence-based medicine: a new approach to teaching the practice of medicine. JAMA 1992;268(17): 2420–5.
2. Chung KC, Swanson JA, Schmitz D, et al. Introducing evidence-based medicine to plastics and reconstructive surgery. Plast Reconstr Surg 2009; 123(4):1385–9.
3. Sackett DL, Rosenberg WM, Gray JA, et al. Evidence-based medicine: what it is and what it isn't. BMJ 1996;312(7023):71–2.
4. Centre for evidence-based medicine. Available at: http://cebm.net. Accessed March 3, 2015.
5. Shaye DA, Tollefson TT, Strong EB. Use of intraoperative computed tomography for maxillofacial reconstructive surgery. JAMA Facial Plast Surg 2015;17(2):113–9.
6. Bray D, Henstrom DK, Cheney ML, et al. Assessing outcomes in facial reanimation: evaluation and validation of the SMILE system for measuring lip excursion during smiling. Arch Facial Plast Surg 2010; 12(5):352–4.
7. Dey JK, Ishii LE, Byrne PJ, et al. The social penalty of facial lesions: new evidence supporting high-quality reconstruction. JAMA Facial Plast Surg 2015;17(2):90–6.
8. Ishii LE. Moving toward objective measurement of facial deformities: exploring a third domain of social perception. JAMA Facial Plast Surg 2015. http://dx.doi.org/10.1001/jamafacial.2015.36.
9. Ishii LE, Rhee JS. Are diagnostic tests useful for nasal valve compromise? Laryngoscope 2013; 123(1):7–8.
10. Graham R, Mancher M, Wolman D, et al. Clinical practice guidelines we can trust. Washington, DC: The National Academies Press; 2011.
11. Rosenfeld R, Piccirillo JF, Chandrasekhar SS, et al. Clinical practice guideline (update): adult sinusitis. Otolaryngol Head Neck Surg 2015;152(2 Suppl): S1–39.

Systematic Review and Meta-Analysis in Facial Plastic Surgery

 CrossMark

Basil Hassouneh, MD[a,b], Michael J. Brenner, MD[c,*]

KEYWORDS

- Systematic review • Meta-analysis • Facial plastic surgery • Rhinoplasty • Rhytidectomy
- Local flap • Reconstruction • Evidence-based medicine

KEY POINTS

- Systematic reviews of the literature involve rigorous methods analogous to primary research studies. Investigators collect, analyze, and interpret data in an explicit, reproducible manner to avoid bias.
- Meta-analysis involves statistical pooling of data derived from multiple studies. To avoid bias in data selection, meta-analyses should be based on an underlying systematic review.
- Systematic reviews and meta-analyses strengthen the evidence base in facial plastic surgery. Functional rhinoplasty, facial reanimation, facial reconstruction, and wound healing are among several areas with potential for enhancing level of evidence.
- In facial plastic surgery, accruing well-designed original studies improves the data set available for systematic reviews and meta-analyses.
- Current challenges include limited numbers of studies, weaknesses of study design/methods, and inconsistency in outcomes and definitions.

INTRODUCTION

Facial plastic and reconstructive surgery is a highly specialized but remarkably diverse specialty, ranging from cosmetic rhinoplasty and facial rejuvenation surgery to craniofacial trauma reconstruction, cleft lip and palate surgery, microvascular surgery, and facial reanimation. In an era of evidence-based medicine, this diversity presents unique challenges and opportunities for facial plastic surgeons. Patients, practitioners, policymakers, and third-party payers all increasingly seek evidence-based answers to specific clinical questions: How prevalent is this clinical problem? What are the risk factors for a particular complication? How effective is one surgical procedure compared with another? Systematic reviews and meta-analyses provide transparent and rigorous summaries of the best available evidence. They are an important addition to the literature because the conclusions play a critical role in developing practice guidelines, identifying gaps in knowledge, defining surgical quality metrics, and allocating resources.

Disclosures: The authors have nothing to disclose.
[a] Department of Otolaryngology – Head and Neck Surgery, University of Toronto, 190 Elizabeth Street - Rm 3S438, Toronto, ON M5G 2N2, Canada; [b] Eye Face Institute, 4789 Yonge Street, Suite 316, Toronto, Ontario M2N 0G3, Canada; [c] Division of Facial Plastic and Reconstructive Surgery, Department of Otolaryngology – Head and Neck Surgery, University of Michigan School of Medicine, 1500 East Medical Center Drive SPC 5312, 1904 Taubman Center, Ann Arbor, MI 48109-5312, USA
* Corresponding author.
E-mail address: mbren@umich.edu

Facial Plast Surg Clin N Am 23 (2015) 273–283
http://dx.doi.org/10.1016/j.fsc.2015.04.001
1064-7406/15/$ – see front matter © 2015 Elsevier Inc. All rights reserved.

WHAT IS A SYSTEMATIC REVIEW

Early efforts to summarize evidence in clinical medicine took the form of narrative expert reviews. They lacked clear structure and were subject to the author's bias in the selection of the literature and the synthesis of the findings. Conversely, the systematic review follows a structured and reproducible process for searching, selecting, and summarizing the available evidence. This process minimizes bias and provides transparent and reliable answers to clinical questions. The process starts with formulating a focused clinical question and is followed by a comprehensive review of the medical literature. Explicit criteria then determine which studies are used to formulate a clinical summary of the findings. Systematic reviews with meta-analyses can summarize the best available evidence to answer many clinical questions in facial plastic surgery.

HOW TO CONDUCT A SYSTEMATIC REVIEW

The systematic review is analogous to primary research in that one reports methods, data collection, and analysis. First, one defines a focused review question and specifies a search strategy of the medical literature that captures most, if not all, of the relevant literature.[1] The review proceeds to identify the eligible studies and evaluate the quality of the available evidence. Frequently, a systematic review is then combined with a meta-analysis, although they are methodologically distinct.

Defining the Research Question

The first, and sometimes most difficult, step is to define the objective of the systematic review. This objective can usually be expressed as a specific clinical question. The acronym PICOT is sometimes used to describe key components of the research question: Population, Intervention, Comparison, Outcome, and Time. It is advisable to survey the available literature to guide the development of a feasible research question. This consideration is particularly relevant in facial plastic surgery, where the small sample size, difficulty of randomizing surgical patients, and the inconsistent outcome measures limit the research data. It is important to determine whether the research question is dealing with cause, diagnosis, intervention, prognosis, or cost. The type of the research question dictates the most suitable study design and the potential biases that may influence findings. For example, when one wants to evaluate if perioperative steroids decrease perioperative edema and ecchymosis following rhinoplasty, the highest quality studies should be randomized

clinical trials (RCTs). However, if the review question is examining which facial nerve outcome scale has the best reliability and validity, the studies are cohorts of patients with facial nerve deficit.

Developing a Search Strategy

Systematic reviews are distinguished from other reviews by the well-structured, explicit, and reproducible search strategy. The strategy is designed based on the PICOT components of the review question. Although the goal is to capture all the relevant studies, increasing the comprehensiveness (or sensitivity) of a search reduces its precision and therefore yields many nonrelevant studies. The search should strike a favorable balance between being comprehensive, yet relevant and manageable. Navigating though databases, such as MEDLINE, EMBASE, or CENTRAL, can be technically demanding, and collaborating with a health care librarian is strongly recommended. Each database has developed specific "controlled vocabulary" and filters to retrieve the studies of interest from millions of publications. It is important that the search is performed in more than one database using controlled vocabulary and regular text words. Filters and limit terms can be added to refine the search, such as a language, publication date, study design, or population age. Although most systematic reviews are limited to the published literature, some review questions call for searching though dissertations, trial registries, meeting abstracts, or even contacting agencies or health providers. This is important in areas were publication bias is thought to heavily influence the results, such as adverse events and complications. Finally, the retrieved articles from several databases and any unpublished articles are merged together in a master library and duplicates removed. **Fig. 1** illustrates the value of a comprehensive search strategy that uses more than one database and possibly includes unpublished results.

Identifying the Evidence

Once the pool of candidate articles has been accumulated, the reviewers then determine which articles meet the defined criteria for inclusion. The inclusion and exclusion criteria should be clearly specified a priori. It is typical for the search to retrieve several hundreds or even thousands of articles that need to be distilled to reach a handful of eligible studies. This process is often done in two stages. First, the reviewers screen the titles and abstracts to identify any potential articles. Subsequently, two independent reviewers evaluate the screened publications using the inclusion and exclusion criteria.

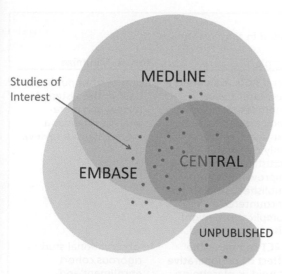

Studies of Interest

MEDLINE

EMBASE

CENTRAL

UNPUBLISHED

Fig. 1. Venn diagram showing the interrelationship of several databases that may be used in a systematic review. Note the spread of data, spanning the three databases and the unpublished data, which is not usually retrievable in electronic searches.

Disagreements between the two reviewers are resolved by consensus or by a third adjudicator (kappa statistical can be provided as a measure of disagreement). This provides validity to the selection process by minimizing bias or arbitrary selection. It is helpful when the reviewers perform piloting to ensure that the selection criteria are clear and reproducible. If the criteria are vague and are heavily influenced by subjective interpretation, there may be substantial disagreements that call into question the reliability (reproducibility) of the selection process. Once the eligible studies are finalized, the data are extracted from each study using standardized data extraction forms. Usually the methodologic details, sample size, and numerical results are summarized into a review table. An example data extraction form is available from the Cochrane collaboration (http://www.cochrane-renal.org/docs/data_extraction_form.doc).

Evaluating Quality of Evidence and Bias

Rigorous quality control is an important feature of the systematic review. The methodologic quality of each included study is evaluated with particular focus on the risk of bias. Bias introduces systematic deviation from the truth and can corrupt the results of the study. Experimental and observational studies alike can be subject to the five classic types of bias: (1) reporting bias, (2) selection bias, (3) performance bias, (4) attrition bias, and (5) detection bias.[2] **Table 1** summarizes these biases and provides practical examples. Reporting (publication) bias refers to a deviation typically toward

favorable results in published studies compared with unpublished studies. Selection bias occurs when each group is selected differently causing incomparable groups with regard to important baseline characteristics and predictors of outcome. In studies of etiology or prognosis, selection bias can lead to a confounding effect. This is a distortion of the association between the exposure and the outcome because the study groups differ with respect to other factors that influence the outcome. Performance bias is a result of major differences in care among groups that influence the outcome. Attrition bias occurs if the rate of withdrawal was unequal between the study groups. Withdrawals from the study lead to incomplete outcome data that influence the analysis. Detection bias is a systematic difference between groups in how the outcome is determined or assessed. There are several instruments developed to evaluate the risk of bias based on the methodologic quality of the study. The QUADAS (quality assessment of diagnostic accuracy studies)[3] and Jadad scale[4] (a brief instrument that evaluates risk of bias in RCTs) are among the commonly used instruments. The risk of bias is dictated by the specifics of the review question. For example, the risk of detection bias (how outcome is evaluated) can range from substantial if the outcome is "soft" (eg, surgeon rating of rhinoplasty outcome) to minimal if the outcome is "hard" (eg, pneumothorax after rib harvest).[5] Accordingly, masking of the individual assessing the outcome is very important in the case of soft outcome but less critical in the case of hard outcome.

WHAT IS A META-ANALYSIS?

Meta-analysis is a statistical method to pool data from two or more studies. This quantitative synthesis aims to answer the research question with greater precision (certainty) and generalizability (external validity) than is possible from individual studies. It can also provide new knowledge that explains the variability observed in the literature or highlight unrecognized aspects of the research question, such as an effect modifier. We highlight a landmark meta-epidemiology by Wood and colleagues[6] that examined 1346 RCTs to compare "double-blind" trials with those without double-blinding. The review demonstrated that lack of blinding was associated with an overall 7% (95% confidence interval, 0–17) exaggeration of treatment effect, which increased to 25% (95% confidence interval, 18–39) in trials with "subjective outcomes." The findings supported the importance of blinding to minimize bias, particularly in trials with subjective outcomes.

Table 1
Summary of five classic types of bias that are evaluated in primary studies

Type of Bias	Definition	Example	How to Minimize
Reporting bias (publication bias)	There is deviation, typically toward favorable results, in published studies compared with unpublished studies.	Several RCTs evaluate if a new laser delivery improves facial aging compared with an existing treatment. Only the trials with statistically significant improvement are published; studies that encountered complications might also be suppressed.	Inclusion of unpublished data in the systematic review and meta-analysis provides a more balanced review.
Selection bias	Each group is selected differently, causing incomparable groups with regard to important baseline characteristics and predictors of outcome.	An RCT compares the effect of perioperative steroid vs placebo on decreasing facial edema after septorhinoplasty. Patients with more extensive osteotomies and bone mobilization were allocated to the treatment group.	In observational studies, rigorous cohort enrollment and adjustment methods, if required. In RCTs, allocation concealment can prevent biased selection.
Performance bias	Substantial differences in care among groups influence the outcome.	A cohort study evaluates if antibiotic use after laser resurfacing decreases the risk of infection. The treating physicians were not masked and were more likely to add topical antibiotic treatment to the control group.	Masking the health care providers to be unaware of patient allocation and treatment.
Attrition bias	The rate of withdrawal is unequal between the study groups, leading to incomplete data that influence the analysis.	A study compares repeated filler injection with placebo. Patients receiving placebo injections were more likely to drop out or not comply with follow-up.	Masking of patients may decrease aspects related to patient perception.
Detection bias	A systematic difference exists between groups in how the outcome is determined or assessed.	A study compares two methods of rhinoplasty using surgeon-based outcome. Surgeons' perception and beliefs influence the evaluation of outcome.	Masking the assessors of outcome to minimize the influence of their beliefs and perceptions.

Relatively few meta-analyses have been conducted in facial plastic surgery, likely because of the demanding methodology and limitations imposed by the available literature. A meta-analysis in the *Aesthetic Surgery Journal* evaluated if perioperative steroids after rhinoplasty minimize edema and ecchymosis.[7] The study included seven RCTs without evaluation of bias or heterogeneity. The statistical pooling failed to use acceptable methods, but rather combined absolute means without forest plot presentation. The authors concluded that "perioperative steroid decreases postoperative edema and ecchymosis associated with rhinoplasty" and made a strong recommendation for "evidence-based guidelines" supporting their use. Recently, a rigorous meta-analysis was completed by the Cochrane group using high-sensitivity literature search and detailed methodologic evaluation of the trials.[8] The review identified nine eligible RCTs examining rhinoplasty, with two trials suitable for meta-analysis. Their review presented full evaluation of bias and heterogeneity; the standardized mean difference was pooled using a fixed-effects model. The authors concluded: "There is limited evidence that high doses of corticosteroids decrease both ecchymosis and edema. The clinical significance of this decrease is unknown, and there is little evidence available regarding the safety of this intervention...Therefore, the current evidence does not support use of corticosteroids as a routine treatment in Facial Plastic Surgery."

HOW TO CONDUCT A META-ANALYSIS

We present a practical framework for understanding and conducting meta-analyses. A complete systematic review is required before starting the meta-analysis. If the systematic review has two or more studies that can be quantitatively combined, then a meta-analysis can be performed. The process requires standardizing the results, evaluating heterogeneity, synthesizing a summary, and finally evaluating robustness (sensitivity analysis). **Table 2** highlights the systematic reviews and meta-analyses retrieved from important journals in facial plastic surgery.

Standardizing the Results

It is important to first understand the type of data under study. Some data are from validated continuous or ordinal scales, such as the Nasal Obstruction Symptom Evaluation scale and the Wrinkle Severity Rating Scale.[9,10] Other outcomes are dichotomous, such as the presence of infection or extrusion of implant. Time-to-event and count variables are unusual in facial plastic surgery but may be encountered in the reporting of rare adverse events or rates. To allow meaningful pooling of the results, the type of outcome needs to be similar across studies. For example, if one study is reporting satisfaction with rhinoplasty as a dichotomous outcome and another study is reporting the satisfaction on an ordinal scale, then these outcomes cannot be simply pooled together. In some circumstances, it might be appropriate to collapse the ordinal scale into a dichotomous scale.

Next, the outcome of interest is extracted from each study using consistent methodology. Relative estimates (odds ratio, relative risk, mean difference) are preferable to absolute estimates of effect size. For continuous data, the mean with standard deviation can be extracted directly. If standard deviation is not reported, it is calculated from the standard error, confidence interval, or P value. Ordinal data can be handled in several ways, depending on the data distribution. Frequently, the ordinal scale is treated as a continuous variable when the scale is large enough and the data exhibit symmetric distribution. Alternatively, the data can be dichotomized or (rarely) maintained as a median with interquartile range. For dichotomous outcomes, the number of positive/negative events can be extracted directly.

Evaluating Heterogeneity

The step of evaluating heterogeneity is critical because it dictates whether data from different studies can be combined. Statistical heterogeneity refers to the interstudy variability of data. Heterogeneity can be evaluated graphically with forest plot (based on the overlap in the confidence intervals) or statistically with a chi-square statistical.[11] Some differences between studies are expected by chance (sampling variation); however, statistically significant heterogeneity should be explored and explained. The variability in clinical factors (population, intervention, and outcome) and the variability in methodologic factors (study design and risk of bias) need to be carefully examined.[12] Only sufficiently similar studies are grouped and meta-analyzed together because combining conflicting results provides misleading estimates and obscures important findings. When heterogeneity cannot be explained, one may opt to use a statistical approach that assumes a distribution of effect (random-effects model). Nonetheless, if the results are widely different or conflicting, it might be more suitable to avoid the pooling of the results and instead provide a qualitative summary. Consider a meta-analysis of Nasal Obstruction Symptom Evaluation scale outcomes following functional rhinoplasty. Some studies may have male patients with a history of trauma, whereas others might be predominantly females with esthetic goals. Heterogeneity arising from such population differences is important to recognize. It is preferable to stratify the studies into separate groups rather than obscuring the difference with inappropriate pooling.

Synthesizing a Summary

Meta-analysis cannot simply "add up" the numerical results of the individual studies as if they all belonged to one big group. Rather, the quantitative synthesis requires appropriate statistical methods.

Table 2
Summary of systematic reviews and meta-analysis retrieved from journals in facial plastic surgery

Author, Year	Scope	Review Question	Outcomes	Conclusions
Wee et al,[13] 2015	Rhinoplasty	Evaluate complications related to autologous rib cartilage rhinoplasty	Nasal complications, donor-site morbidity, and revision surgery	Long-term complications and donor-site morbidity rates associated with autologous rib cartilage use in rhinoplasty were low. Because of limitations future studies are needed.
Paleri et al,[18] 2014	Microvascular	Evaluated impact of vascularized tissue on fistula rate after laryngectomy reconstruction	Fistula rate	Flap reconstruction/reinforcement with vascularized tissue reduced their risk of pharyngocutaneous fistula by approximately one-third.
Rhee et al,[19] 2014	Rhinoplasty	Define symptomatic, normative, and postoperative values for nasal obstruction	Nasal obstruction assessed with VAS and NOSE	VAS and NOSE can be used as a clinically meaningful measure of successful surgical outcomes.
da Silva et al,[8] 2014	Perioperative	To determine the effects, including safety, of perioperative administration of corticosteroids for preventing complications following facial plastic surgery in adults	Ecchymosis and edema	Limited evidence that corticosteroids decrease ecchymosis and edema. There is little evidence regarding the safety of this intervention.
Cheung et al,[20] 2013	Trauma	Determine safety and efficacy of endoscopic management of isolated orbital floor fractures	Resolution of diplopia and enophthalmos, postoperative complications	Reconstruction of orbital floor fractures through an endoscopic approach seems to be safe and effective.
Morris & Kellman,[21] 2014	Trauma (antibiotics)	Studied role of prophylactic antibiotics in the management of facial fractures	Postoperative infection rate	Risk of infection in patients with mandibular fractures is reduced with use of prophylactic antibiotics from time of injury to completion of the perioperative course.

Source	Topic	Objective	Outcome Measures	Conclusion
Picavet et al,[22] 2011	BDD	Assessment of screening tools for BDD in cosmetic surgery setting	BDD questionnaire–dermatology version, dysmorphic concern questionnaire	Despite high prevalence of BDD in cosmetic surgery, little is known about these tools in the cosmetic surgery setting. Further research is needed on the prevalence of BDD in cosmetic surgery and impact of BDD on treatment outcomes.
André et al,[23] 2009	Rhinoplasty	Studied the relationship between subjective and objective evaluation of the nasal airway	Rhinomanometry, acoustic rhinometry, patient-reported outcomes	Patients' subjective nasal obstruction does not correlate well with rhinomanometry and acoustic rhinometry. There is thus little evidence for routine use of rhinomanometry or acoustic rhinometry for quantifying surgical results in clinical rhinologic practice.
Spielmann et al,[24] 2009	Rhinoplasty	Evaluate surgical treatment strategies for nasal valve collapse	Subjective symptom relief, cosmetic outcome, objective measurements of nasal airway patency	No randomized controlled trials on nasal valve surgery were identified. Reporting of long-term outcomes is limited. There is uncertainty regarding evidence base for choice of specific technique and duration of benefit.
Nash et al,[25] 2010	Trauma/facial nerve	Evaluate impact of early surgical intervention vs steroid administration/observation	House-Brackmann scale	The available evidence does not clearly indicate whether surgical vs nonsurgical intervention achieves most favorable outcome for facial paralysis after trauma.
Rhee & McMullin,[26] 2008	Measurement	Identify outcome instruments specific for facial plastic surgery interventions and conditions	Outcome instruments validation	Validated outcome measures are available for common facial plastic surgery conditions. Challenges remain in harmonizing and standardizing the different measures to reach clinically

(continued on next page)

Table 2
(continued)

Author, Year	Scope	Review Question	Outcomes	Conclusions
				meaningful assessments of outcomes.
Rhee et al,[27] 2008	Rhinoplasty	Critical review of evidence supporting functional rhinoplasty or nasal valve repair	Validated patient-reported outcome measures	Level 4 evidence supports the efficacy of functional rhinoplasty for treatment of nasal obstruction arising from nasal valve collapse. Further studies with standardized objective outcome measures and comparison cohorts are needed.
Leventhal et al,[28] 2006	Wound healing	Determine treatments that can improve keloid and hypertrophic scars	Assessment of keloid and hypertrophic scars	Most treatments for keloidal and hypertrophic scarring offer minimal likelihood of improvement.
Koch & Perkins,[29] 2002	Rhytidectomy/laser	Evaluate the safety of combining carbon dioxide laser resurfacing with full-face rhytidectomy	Rate of postoperative complications	Simultaneous rhytidectomy and carbon dioxide laser resurfacing can safely provide a dual cosmetic benefit for aesthetic rejuvenation.

The journals *JAMA Facial Plastic Surgery, Laryngoscope, JAMA Otolaryngology,* and *Otolaryngology – Head & Neck Surgery* were searched using publication type limit to "review," "systematic review," or "meta-analysis." Cochrane library was also searched for related reviews. The titles and abstracts were first screened, and then two reviewers independently identified eligible studies (systematic review or meta-analysis in facial plastic surgery). Subsequently, the data were extracted from each eligible study using standardized form and summarized.

Abbreviations: BDD, body dysmorphic disorder; NOSE, Nasal Obstruction Symptom Evaluation scale; VAS, visual analog scale.

Data from Refs. 8,13,18–29

There are two main approaches to combine individual estimates: the fixed-effects model assumes that the effect is similar between studies, whereas the random-effects model assumes a distribution of effect size across studies. When there is no heterogeneity among studies, both the fixed-effects and the random-effects models provide identical pooled estimation. Nonetheless, when there is significant heterogeneity, the confidence interval for the pooled estimation is wider (thus statistical significance more conservative) with the random-effects compared with the fixed-effects model. The results are then summarized graphically in a forest plot that provides the individual and the pooled estimations with the corresponding confidence intervals. **Fig. 2** presents a conceptual schematic of a forest plot from a meta-analysis. Such presentations are beginning to find application in the facial plastic surgery literature, as in a recent comprehensive report examining rates of warping, resorption, infection, and displacement associated with rib cartilage use in rhinoplasty.[13]

Several statistical methods have been developed for meta-analysis.[14] The fixed-effects model is most commonly performed with inverse variance method, where the weight given to each study corresponds to the inverse of the variance (reciprocal of the standard error squared). Thus, larger studies have more weight because they have smaller standard errors. When the sample size is small or the event rate is low, the inverse variance method leads to a poor estimation, and the Mantel-Haenszel method is preferred. Peto method is another modification of inverse variance that uses observed and expected statistics to estimate log odds ratio. It can only be used with odds ratio but has the advantage of not requiring correction for zero cells (groups without events). A random-effects model can sometimes be used to accommodate the variability.[15] The model assumes a lack of knowledge about why an effect varies and considers that the effect has a distribution. The center of the distribution describes the average effect, whereas the width represents the degree of variability.

Facial plastic surgery presents some challenges for meta-analysis. First, as in other surgical fields, RCTs are sparse and most of the evidence is formed with small sample size observational studies of variable methodology. Second, despite some recent contributions, patient-centered outcome measures are relatively underdeveloped without clear consensus in reporting. The grading of outcome and severity for facial nerve deficit illustrates the dilemma. A recent systematic review identified 19 different scales; almost all scales had severe limitations in several measurement aspects and unclear correlation with patient's quality-of-life.[16] In such cases with marked variability in the methodology and outcome assessment, individual-level data meta-analysis can offer a suitable solution.[17] For example, if individual studies of facial nerve outcome can provide sufficient descriptive details for each case, this may facilitate rescore in a standardized scale to allow individual-level data pooling of the results.

Evaluating Robustness (Sensitivity Analysis)

Completing a systematic review and meta-analysis requires a sequence of decisions. Although the process is structured, some steps might be arbitrary, based on assumption, or subject to opinion. This can make the results of the meta-analysis vulnerable. A sensitivity analysis is a repeat of the meta-analysis with an alternative decision or approach; it aims to evaluate the robustness of the results in the face of specific vulnerabilities. For example, the eligibility of some studies might be subject to opinion because of unclear methodologic reporting. Here the sensitivity analysis might repeat the meta-analysis with only the "certainly" eligible studies included. Similarly, the assumption of insignificant heterogeneity might not be clear, and the sensitivity analysis can repeat the statistical pooling with a random-effects method. When the results of the sensitivity

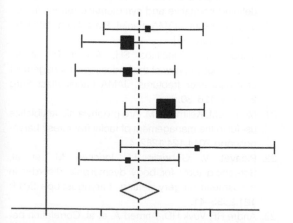

Fig. 2. Appearance of a generic forest plot, depicting distribution and weight of constituent studies included in meta-analysis. In the example shown, odds ratios from six (fictitious) studies are depicted, with the size of each *square* proportional to the weight of the study in the meta-analysis. The *horizontal lines* reflect the confidence intervals of individual studies. The *diamond* represents a summary measure, the *width of the diamond* reflects the confidence interval, and the *solid vertical line* corresponds to no effect.

analysis align with the results of the primarily analysis, the findings are robust. Nonetheless, if the difference is substantial then the synthesis is sensitive to specific assumptions, and this should be considered when formulating conclusions and recommendations.

SUMMARY

Systematic reviews and meta-analysis have a well-established role in summarizing the best available evidence to answer a specific clinical question. They are the supporting foundation for clinical guidelines and policy decisions. Nonetheless, this valuable research continues to be underused in facial plastic surgery. This situation is likely caused by the technical challenges imposed by the current state of the literature, but also by the demanding aspects of the methodology. A collaborative effort is required to make high-quality systematic reviews and meta-analyses achievable.

REFERENCES

1. Liberati A, Altman DG, Tetzlaff J, et al. The PRISMA statement for reporting systematic reviews and meta-analyses of studies that evaluate healthcare interventions: explanation and elaboration. BMJ 2009; 339:b2700.
2. Paradis C. Bias in surgical research. Ann Surg 2008; 248:180–8.
3. Whiting PR, Rutjes A, Dinnes J, et al. Development and validation of methods for assessing the quality of diagnostic accuracy studies. Health Technol Assess 2004;8:1–234.
4. Jadad AR, Moore RA, Carroll D, et al. Assessing the quality of reports of randomized clinical trials: is blinding necessary? Control Clin Trials 1996;17:1–12.
5. Hassouneh BG, Welch HG. Blinding who from what?. In: Berger VW, Zhang XC, editors. Important considerations for clinical trial methodologies. London: Future Science Ltd; 2013. p. 62–77.
6. Wood L, Egger M, Gluud LL, et al. Empirical evidence of bias in treatment effect estimates in controlled trials with different interventions and outcomes: meta-epidemiological study. BMJ 2008;336:601–5.
7. Hatef DA, Ellsworth WA, Allen JN, et al. Perioperative steroids for minimizing edema and ecchymosis after rhinoplasty: a meta-analysis. Aesthet Surg J 2011;31:648–57.
8. da Silva EM, Hochman B, Ferreira LM. Perioperative corticosteroids for preventing complications following facial plastic surgery. Cochrane Database Syst Rev 2014;(6):CD009697.
9. Day DJ, Littler CM, Swift RW, et al. The wrinkle severity rating scale: a validation study. Am J Clin Dermatol 2004;5:49–52.
10. Stewart MG, Witsell DL, Smith TL, et al. Development and validation of the Nasal Obstruction Symptom Evaluation (NOSE) scale. Otolaryngol Head Neck Surg 2004;130:157–63.
11. Higgins JP, Thompson SG. Quantifying heterogeneity in a meta-analysis. Stat Med 2002;21:1539–58.
12. Thompson SG. Why sources of heterogeneity in meta-analysis should be investigated. BMJ 1994; 309:1351–5.
13. Wee JH, Park MH, Oh S, et al. Complications associated with autologous rib cartilage use in rhinoplasty: a meta-analysis. JAMA Facial Plast Surg 2015;17:49–55.
14. Thompson SG, Higgins JP. How should meta-regression analyses be undertaken and interpreted? Stat Med 2002;21:1559–73.
15. Riley RD, Higgins JP, Deeks JJ. Interpretation of random effects meta-analyses. BMJ 2011;342: d549.
16. Fattah A, Gurusinghe A, Gavilan J, et al. Facial nerve grading instruments: systematic review of the literature and suggestion for uniformity. Plast Reconstr Surg 2015;135(2):569–79.
17. Riley RD, Lambert PC, Abo-Zaid G. Meta-analysis of individual participant data: rationale, conduct, and reporting. BMJ 2010;340:c221.
18. Paleri V, Drinnan M, van den Brekel MW, et al. Vascularized tissue to reduce fistula following salvage total laryngectomy: a systematic review. Laryngoscope 2014;124:1848–53.
19. Rhee JS, Sullivan CD, Frank DO, et al. A systematic review of patient-reported nasal obstruction scores: defining normative and symptomatic ranges in surgical patients. JAMA Facial Plast Surg 2014;16: 219–25 [quiz: 32].
20. Cheung K, Voineskos SH, Avram R, et al. A systematic review of the endoscopic management of orbital floor fractures. JAMA Facial Plast Surg 2013;15:126–30.
21. Morris LM, Kellman RM. Are prophylactic antibiotics useful in the management of facial fractures? Laryngoscope 2014;124:1282–4.
22. Picavet V, Gabriels L, Jorissen M, et al. Screening tools for body dysmorphic disorder in a cosmetic surgery setting. Laryngoscope 2011; 121:2535–41.
23. André RF, Vuyk HD, Ahmed A, et al. Correlation between subjective and objective evaluation of the nasal airway. A systematic review of the highest level of evidence. Clin Otolaryngol 2009;34:518–25.
24. Spielmann PM, White PS, Hussain SS. Surgical techniques for the treatment of nasal valve collapse: a systematic review. Laryngoscope 2009;119:1281–90.
25. Nash JJ, Friedland DR, Boorsma KJ, et al. Management and outcomes of facial paralysis from intratemporal blunt trauma: a systematic review. Laryngoscope 2010;120(Suppl 4):S214.

26. Rhee JS, McMullin BT. Outcome measures in facial plastic surgery: patient-reported and clinical efficacy measures. Arch Facial Plast Surg 2008;10:194–207.

27. Rhee JS, Arganbright JM, McMullin BT, et al. Evidence supporting functional rhinoplasty or nasal valve repair: a 25-year systematic review. Otolaryngol Head Neck Surg 2008;139:10–20.

28. Leventhal D, Furr M, Reiter D. Treatment of keloids and hypertrophic scars: a meta-analysis and review of the literature. Arch Facial Plast Surg 2006;8:362–8.

29. Koch BB, Perkins SW. Simultaneous rhytidectomy and full-face carbon dioxide laser resurfacing: a case series and meta-analysis. Arch Facial Plast Surg 2002;4:227–33.

Skin Care

Amelia Clark, MD, Jill L. Hessler, MD*

KEYWORDS

- Photoaging • Retinoid acid • Sunscreen • Cosmeceutical • Sun damage

KEY POINTS

- Photoaging can be minimized or delayed with proper use of sun protection.
- Retinoids can reverse some of the signs of aging when used consistently.
- Vitamins applied topically can minimize damage from sun exposure and also act as antioxidants to limit environmental damage.
- The SPF system may underestimate the deleterious effects on the skin by neglecting the contributions of ultraviolet A radiation.
- Human studies of topically applied antioxidants are limited, but early work suggests they may have a protective effect against cellular changes resulting from photodamage.

Aging skin is among the most common patient concerns in a facial plastic surgery practice. Ultraviolet (UV)-induced damage expedites the pace of intrinsic aging, resulting in many of the visible signs of aging, such as rough skin texture, pigmentation irregularities, fine and deep wrinkling, and inelasticity. Primary prevention of UV and environmental damage with proper skin care and the use of sunscreen are critical. There is great interest in topically applied products to reverse or delay the visible signs of photoaging. There is an extraordinarily diverse array of prescription and cosmeceutical products available for the consumer. This article discusses the most common topically applied agents for photoaging, reviewing their mechanisms and supporting evidence.

SUNSCREEN

UV irradiation leads to the production of reactive oxygen species and activation of intracellular signaling pathways that result in an increase in inflammatory mediators. These mediators interfere with synthesis of dermal collagens and trigger synthesis of enzymes that degrade the extracellular matrix. This effect is compounded by UV damage to the mitochondrial genome, resulting in double-stranded breaks that affect the mitochondrial ability to produce energy for the cell and lead to further accumulation of reactive oxygen species. Moreover, chronic UV irradiation modifies local immunoregulation and cell survival, leading to impairment of intrinsic cancer surveillance.[1] Both UVA and UVB spectrums are implicated in photodamage. UVB photons are on average 1000 times more energetic than UVA photons, making them a major contributor to photoaging and photocarcinogenesis. However, UVA is found in up to 10 times greater abundance in sunlight, and has greater depth of penetration into the dermis compared with UVB, giving it a possibly even greater role in photoaging.[2] The visible effects of chronic long-term UV exposure are well-understood. The facial skin of females living in regions exposed to higher UV had significantly more and longer wrinkles, more and larger hyperpigmented spots, rougher surface texture, and more yellow discoloration based on computer analysis than women living at lower UV levels.[3] Topical application of photoprotective agents significantly

Disclosure: Consultant Allergan, Galderma (J.L. Hessler); Nothing to disclose (A. Clark).
Otolaryngology, Head and Neck Surgery, Stanford University, 801 Welch Road, Stanford, CA 94035, USA
* Corresponding author.
E-mail address: jillhesslermd@gmail.com

Facial Plast Surg Clin N Am 23 (2015) 285–295
http://dx.doi.org/10.1016/j.fsc.2015.04.002
1064-7406/15/$ – see front matter

reduces the lifetime UV exposure compared with nonuse, with regular daily use beginning early in life being the most important factor.[4] A randomized, controlled Australian study of 903 adults investigated the effect of daily use of a broad-spectrum sunscreen versus discretionary use and found that daily sunscreen use reduces the signs of skin aging based on skin surface replicas (level I evidence).[5] Skin surface replicas were made from the back of the left hand by using a silicone-based impression material. These replicas were then graded by experienced evaluators who were blinded to their treatment group, and assessed based on severity of skin changes. This study found good intragrader and intergrader reliability.

There are 2 main categories of topically applied sunscreens: organic (previously called chemical) and inorganic (previously called physical). Organic sunscreens absorb UV irradiation, converting it to heat and thereby preventing its untoward effects in the skin. These compounds are typically not visible when applied and are therefore widely used. In contrast, inorganic sunscreens contain particles such as zinc oxide or titanium dioxide that reflect photons away from the skin. The earlier generations of inorganic sunscreens were less cosmetically desirable because their large particle size resulted in a visible and comedogenic coating on the skin. Newer iterations have micronized or nanosized the active particles, resulting in improved cosmetic appearance and alteration of the spectral absorption profile.[6] The protection provided by sunscreen agents is traditionally quantified by SPF, or sun protection factor. This measure is defined as the minimal erythemal dose in sunscreen-protected skin divided by the minimal erythemal dose in non–sunscreen-protected skin. As UVB is the overwhelmingly greater contributing factor to sunburn than UVA, the SPF system was created to indicate the level of UVB protection. Thus, there is concern that the SPF system may underestimate the deleterious effects on the skin by neglecting the contributions of UVA radiation. Furthermore, the use of skin erythema as a surrogate for the more important underlying cellular alterations and local immunomodulation is called into question.

New awareness of the effects of UVA and its underrepresentation in current labeling systems prompted the US Food and Drug Administration (FDA) in 2011 to publish new guidelines directing the labeling and effectiveness testing for sunscreens. This ruling outlined the testing standards for coverage against both UVA and UVB for sunscreen to carry a label of "broad spectrum." Also, this ruling for the first time provided permission for broad-spectrum sunscreen with SPF of 15 or greater to carry the claim to decrease skin cancer and early skin aging.[7] One important issue addressed in the recent ruling is that there is no maximum allowable SPF label. Companies market sunscreens with SPF exceeding 100, which may provide consumers with a false sense of protection, resulting in prolonged UV exposure and failure to reapply sunscreen as directed. There is thus a recommendation by the FDA to cap the maximum SPF label at 50+, because there is not sufficient evidence to support increasing efficacy beyond SPF 50.[8] There is not currently a UVA rating system in the United States, although a 5-star UVA protection rating system has been recommended for industry use in the European Union.

RETINOIDS

Topical retinoids as a treatment for photoaging have the most extensive evidence-based support in the literature and, not surprisingly, has been widely adopted in clinical practice. Available topical retinoids include retinol, retinaldehyde, tretinoin (retinoic acid), isotretinoin, tazarotene, and adapalene. Tazarotene and adapalene are synthetic retinoinds.

Photodamage expedites the natural aging process resulting in skin discoloration, roughness, and wrinkles, the appearance of which can be improved with the use of retinoids. Retinoids act via a tretinoin-specific gene transcription factor, suggesting that retinoids leverage their effect on the skin through regulated gene expression.[9] On a molecular level, retinoids bind to specific retinoic acid receptors, which serve as ligand-dependent transcription factors that regulate a diverse array of mediators to increase epidermal integrity and modulate the production of procollagen.[10] As reviewed by Fisher and Voorhees in 1996,[11] retinoid acts in vivo by inducing keratinocyte proliferation and modulating their differentiation, thereby increasing epidermal thickness, even by as much as 40% in some studies (compared with 10% in controls).[12] This effect occurs regardless of topical or oral administration, which argues against a previously held belief that retinoid effect was mitigated solely through its irritant effect on the skin. Histologically, topical tretinoin has been shown to result in epidermal hyperplasia, compaction of the stratum corneum, and restoration of cell polarity.[13] In addition to modulating cellular proliferation, some of the effects of retinoids may be mediated through collagen synthesis. Dermal collagen is central for providing resiliency to the skin, and its regulation and synthesis is an important component in the mechanism of the effect of tretinoin on photoaging.

In a study by Talwar and colleagues,[14] photoaged forearm skin was significantly lower in types I and III collagen compared with sun-protected underarm and buttock skin in a dose-dependent manner. A follow-up study demonstrated that 10 to 12 months of tretinoin use for photoaging resulted in a restoration of collagen I staining by 80% above baseline, compared with a 14% reduction in the control group.[15]

Early studies provided immediate promise for the use of retinoids. In a randomized, double-blind, placebo-controlled study from 1988, Weiss and colleagues[16] enrolled 30 participants for a 16-week study during which 0.1% tretinoin was applied to 1 forearm, and a vehicle cream that did not contain tretinoin was applied to the other (level II evidence; only a single rater was utilized). One-half of the patients applied tretinoin to the face and the other half vehicle alone. Improvement in photoaging was reported in all of the treated forearms and in 14 of 15 patients who used tretinoin on the face, based on expert grading of fine and course wrinkling, tactile roughness, and telangiectasia. All parameters except telangiectasia showed improvement, and there was a reduction in the color of solar-induced freckles and lentigines, although not in the absolute lesion number. Skin biopsy specimens were also taken from the forearm, and demonstrated an increase in epidermal thickness and number of mitotic figures as well as an improved organization of the stratum corneum in the tretinoin treated group. This study also correlated clinical changes with histologic outcomes, and noted a significant increase in epidermal thickness and granular layer thickness, a higher mitotic index, and a compaction of the stratum corneum in the treated skin versus vehicle alone (Fig. 1).

Small, early studies such as this were soon reinforced by larger multicenter trials, which have formed a strong evidence base for the efficacy of retinoic acid. A study of 251 patients compared topical tretinoin at concentrations of 0.05% and 0.01% versus vehicle control with outcome measure being improvement in photoaging based on a defined 9-point severity scale and histologic features on punch biopsy (level I evidence).[17] This study demonstrated a significant improvement in photoaging score in the 0.05% group, which was supported by histologic changes, including increased epidermal thickness, decreased melanin content, and stratum corneum compaction. Notable side effects included erythema, peeling, burning, and stinging, which were more notable in the group treated with the higher concentration. A follow-up study from 1992 focused on the dose-related efficacy in comparing topical tretinoin at 0.05%, 0.01%, and 0.001% versus vehicle alone in a multicenter study of 296 patients (level I evidence).[18] This study demonstrated that use of tretinoin 0.05% resulted in an improvement in overall severity of photodamage that increased with duration of use from 12 to 24 weeks, whereas 0.01% and 0.001% tretinoin were not different from vehicle alone in overall skin improvement (Figs. 2 and 3). Recently, a 2-year, multicenter, double-blind, placebo-controlled trial of topical tretinoin 0.05% versus vehicle demonstrated the long-term efficacy of topical retinoic acid use, citing a significant improvement in fine and course wrinkling, mottled hyperpigmentation, and sallowness (level I evidence).[19]

One consistent element across multiple studies of the various forms of topical retinoids is the occurrence of skin irritation, which varies slightly by type of retinoid and concentration used. Irritation can be characterized by redness, burning, peeling, and stinging, and typically abates with increasing duration of use. The widespread incidence of skin irritation underscores the importance of a proper skin care regimen in tandem with the use of topical retinoids. Most skin irritation can be alleviated by a regimen of daily moisturizer and sunscreen use. A several day hiatus from application may also alleviate some of these unwanted side effects. Proper sun protection is essential because retinoids are photosensitizers and can increase the risks associated with sun exposure.

In response to this high incidence of skin irritation with topical tretinoin use, a recent single-blinded study of 24 patients compared the efficacy of topical 0.05% retinoic acid versus 20 mg oral isotretinoin for the treatment of photoaging (level I evidence). After 6 months of every-other-day treatment, no differences were noted between the groups' outcomes, including patient-reported and photographic improvement in skin appearance and quality-of-life metrics. Histologic and immunohistochemical analyses showed similar increase in epidermal thickness and increase in dermal collagen. Adverse effects of oral isotretinoin included mild chelitis, but there were no differences in biochemical safety metrics, including liver function, lipid profile, blood count, or fasting glucose. This suggests that oral isotretinoin as a treatment for photoaging could be considered for the correct candidate patient lacking individual risk factors who demonstrates an intolerance to topical retinoid application.[20]

The cosmeceutical market is a billion-dollar industry, and many natural vitamin A derivatives are available without a prescription. Although there is a large body of literature to support the efficacy of

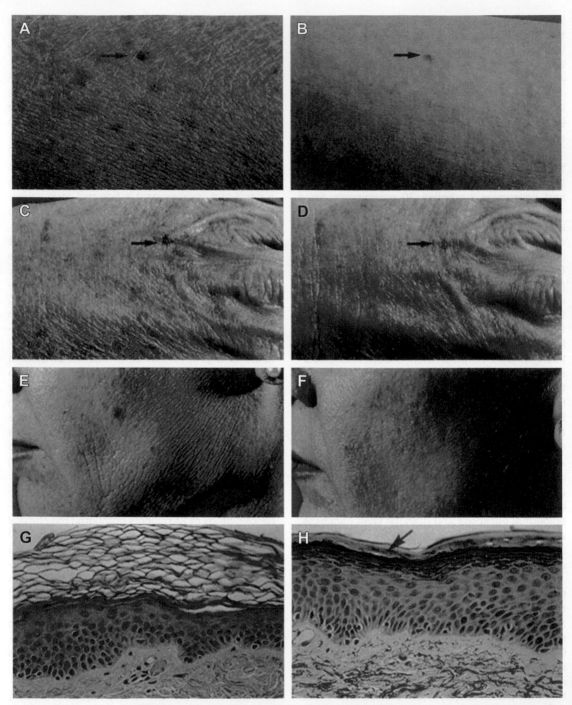

Fig. 1. Left forearm before therapy (*A*) and after 16 weeks of therapy (*B*) with 0.1% tretinoin cream. Note reduction in fine wrinkling and fading of solar induced freckles following therapy. Arrow denotes same freckle before and after treatment. Left hand of patient before therapy (*C*) and after 16 weeks of therapy (*D*). Note increased pinkness and reduced fine wrinkling after treatment with topical tretinoin, as well as fading of dark lentigo (*arrow*). Left cheek of patient before therapy (*E*) and after 16 weeks of therapy (*F*). Note reduction in fine wrinkling and occurrence of pinkness. Forearm skin from same patient before therapy (*G*; stain: hematoxylin and eosin, original magnification ×63) and after 16 weeks of tretinoin therapy (*H*; stain: Movat pentachrome, original magnification ×63) demonstrating glycosaminoglycan-like material (*arrow*) within compacted stratum corneum. Note change in morphology of stratum corneum, normalization of epidermal morphology, and increase in epidermal thickness. (*From* Weiss JS, Ellis CN, Headington JT, et al. Topical tretinoin improves photoaged skin: a double-blind vehicle-controlled study. JAMA 1988;259:530; with permission.)

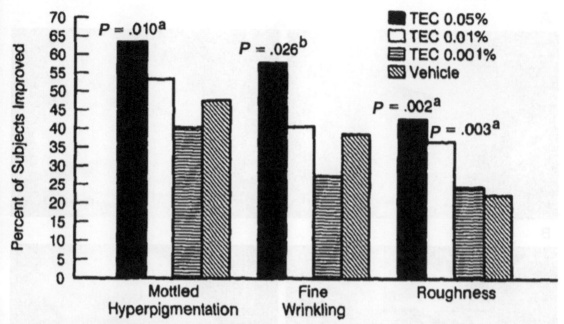

Fig. 2. Improvement in photodamage with varying dosages of tretinoin. Investigator evaluations of mottled hyperpigmentation, fine wrinkling, and roughness after 24 weeks of therapy with varying concentrations of tretinoin and vehicle control. Only 0.05% tretinoin demonstrated statistically significant improvements over control. [a] Statistically significant compared with vehicle. [b] Marginally statistically significant compared with vehicle. (*From* Olsen EA, Katz HI, Levine N, et al. Tretinoin emollient cream: a new therapy for photodamaged skin. J Am Acad Dermatol 1992;26:221; with permission.)

topical tretinoin use in the management of photoaging, scientific evidence to support many of the claims advertised for over-the-counter products is lacking. A review of the available body of evidence for cosmeceutical retinoids demonstrated that the most effective cosmeceutical vitamin A derivative was retinaldehyde, as supported by several large studies that showed improvement in fine and deep wrinkles. Several small, subjective clinical trials demonstrated possible benefit in the use of retinol for photoaging. This review found no significant evidence to support the use of topical retinyl-acetate and retinyl-palmitate.[21]

ALPHA HYDROXY ACIDS

Alpha hydroxy acids are organic acids that have been in use in clinical practice since first described in 1974 by Van Scott and Yu.[22] The most recognizable compounds in this class include glycolic acid, lactic acid, and salicylic acid. Glycolic acid was the first compound in this class to be recognized, but recently a new generation of alpha hydroxyl acids called polyhydroxy acids or polyhydroxy bionic acids have been found to achieve similar effects in photoaging while minimizing irritant side effects. Alpha hydroxy acids modify cell turnover and alter the extracellular matrix by a number of mechanisms, including increasing collagen synthesis by

fibroblasts.[23] In a study of 17 subjects with moderate to severe photodamaged skin, 25% glycolic, lactic, or citric acid was applied to one forearm, and placebo lotion was applied to the other for 6 months (level II evidence).[24] Two-layer skin thickness increased by 25% after treatment with alpha hydroxy acids, along with an increase in collagen and mucopolysaccharide density. In another study from 2001, photodamaged skin was treated with topical 20% glycolic acid lotion (pH 4.3) or a lotion control (pH 3.9) applied twice daily for 3 months, then evaluated histologically and by Northern blot from a skin biopsy specimen (level III evidence). The glycolic acid–treated skin demonstrated increased epidermal thickness, levels of hyaluronic acid within the epidermis and dermis, and collagen gene expression.[25] Even small changes in the amount of dermal glycosaminoglycans can effect massive improvements in the capacity for skin hydration, thereby dramatically affecting texture and appearance, therefore reversing some of the signs of photoaging.

ANTIOXIDANTS
Vitamin C

The skin is subject to great oxidative stressors, such as smoking, pollution, and sunlight, with UV damage being a potent generator of reactive

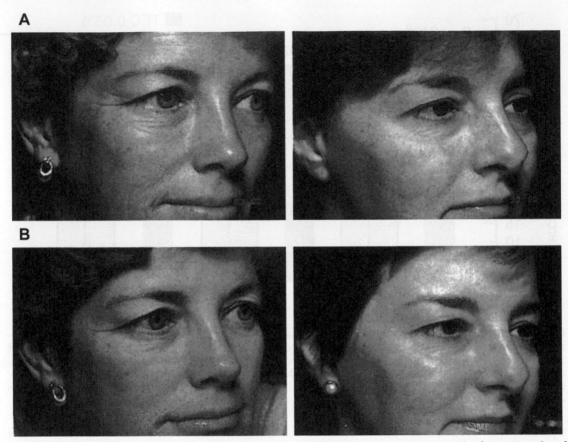

Fig. 3. Left and right: pretreatment appearance (*A*), and posttreatment appearance (*B*) after 24 weeks of tretinoin emollient cream 0.05%. Both subjects were graded by investigator as having an excellent response at week 24. (*From* Olsen EA, Katz HI, Levine N, et al. Tretinoin emollient cream: a new therapy for photodamaged skin. J Am Acad Dermatol 1992;26:218; with permission.)

oxygen species. Given that antioxidants are depleted in the process of their protecting skin from oxidative stress, it is reasonable to improve their reservoir in the skin via topical application. Vitamin C, or ascorbic acid, is prevalent in the extracellular matrix of the skin, where it acts as a scavenger of free radicals. It has also been described as having antiinflammatory properties, given its effect in reducing skin erythema after laser resurfacing.[26] The level of ascorbic acid in the epidermis decreases with age.[27] Most important, ascorbic acid is an essential cofactor for the enzymes lysyl and prolyl hydroxylase, which are required for types I and III collagen synthesis. Indeed, the presence of ascorbic acid has been shown to enhance the transcription of types I and III collagen genes by 4- and 3.4-fold, respectively.[28] In addition to this effect on stimulating transcription of collagen genes, ascorbic acid also decreases the rate of collagen degradation by reducing the production of matrix metalloproteinase.[29]

Several studies have investigated the effects of topical application of ascorbate compounds with doses ranging from 3% to 17%. In a randomized, double-blind, vehicle-controlled, split-face study, 19 patients applied 3% ascorbic acid and vehicle serum to one-half of the face over a 3-month period (level II evidence). Significant improvement was noted in facial wrinkles, roughness, skin laxity, and sallowness as measured by evaluation of standardized photographs and a computer-based analysis of skin surface replicas that digitally analyzed and quantified surface features.[30] This study demonstrated improvement in clinical assessment, computer image analysis of surface replicas, and patient-reported outcomes, but may be limited by a small sample size (**Fig. 4**). Another double-blind, split-face study of 10 patients used topical application of 10% ascorbic acid versus vehicle control, and demonstrated a significant improvement in clinical scoring of perioral and cheek wrinkles at the end of the 90-day study. Several patients in this study underwent

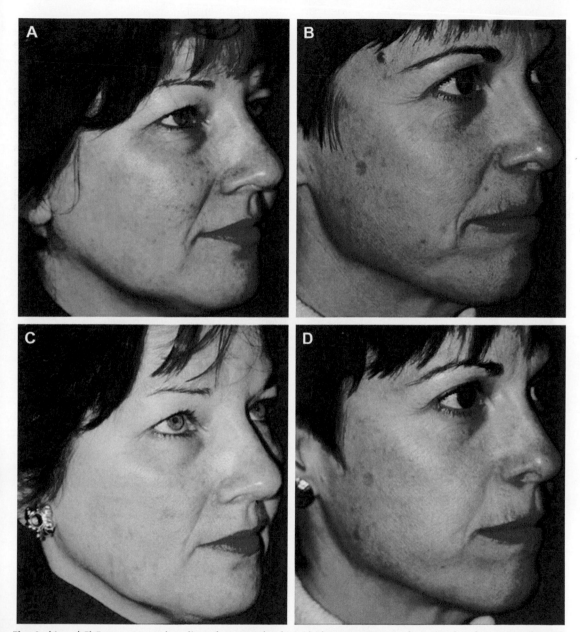

Fig. 4. (*A* and *B*) Pretreatment baseline photographs. (*C* and *D*) Posttreatment photographs after 3-month application of topical ascorbic acid preparation. Note improvement in the periorbital crows feet region and in overall skin texture and tone. (*From* Traikovich SS. Use of topical ascorbic acid and its effects on photodamaged skin topography. Arch Otolaryngol Head Neck Surg 1999;125:1094; with permission.)

biopsy to obtain histology sections, which demonstrated an increase in the amount of collagen in the patients who demonstrated clinical improvement (level II evidence given limited sample size).[31] Last, a double-blind, randomized trial of 20 patients using topical application of 5% ascorbic acid versus vehicle control demonstrated a reduction in facial photoaging by dermatologist grading, as well as an improvement in skin texture on surface replica analysis and improvement in histologic organization collagen and elastin (level I evidence; correlates systematically scored clinical outcomes with histologic analytics).[32] There are some data from animal studies that suggest that vitamin C may also have photoprotective properties. When topically applied, ascorbic acid protected skin from UVB and UVA injury[33] and reducing UVB-induced immunosuppression.[34]

Topical use of ascorbic acid has been shown to be effective in reducing the visible effects of photoaging; however, product stability and skin delivery remain problematic. The products are light sensitive and therefore are generally sold in dark bottles. It is recommended to keep the products in a cabinet and not on a counter to limit the exposure to light. Vitamin C and its derivatives are also extremely oxygen sensitive and degrade rapidly. The oxidation that occurs will manifest as an orange–brown discoloration of the serum. Moreover, the penetration of ascorbic acid across the skin is very poor, making production of a stable product even more challenging.

Vitamin E

Vitamin E is an oil-soluble antioxidant, of which the 2 main classes are tocopherols and tocotrienols, with alpha tocopherol being the major form in humans. Vitamin E is delivered to the stratum corneum by sebaceous glands, where it acts to absorb oxidative environmental stress and is thereby depleted. Several animal studies have demonstrated potential photoprotective effects of vitamin E application, but studies in humans are still forthcoming. There is an important synergistic effect between vitamins E and C; it is through a complex network of redox reactions

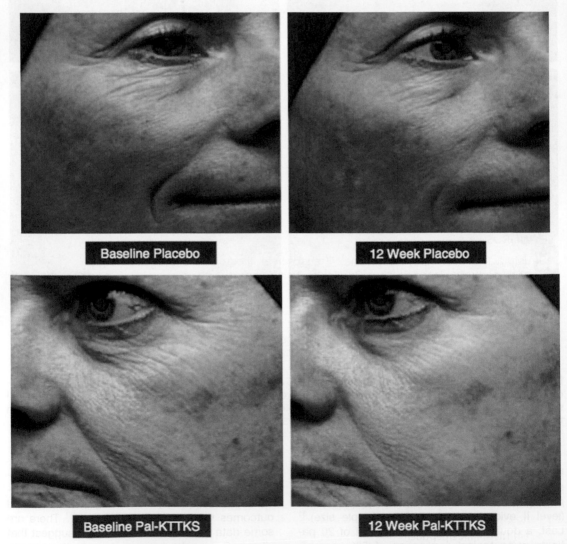

Baseline Placebo   **12 Week Placebo**

Baseline Pal-KTTKS   **12 Week Pal-KTTKS**

Fig. 5. Effect of placebo versus palmitoyl-lysine-threonine-threonine-lysine-serine (pal-KTTKS) peptide formulation after 12 weeks of topical treatment. Note improvement in fine lines and wrinkles in the patient treated with pal-KTTS versus control. (*From* Robinson LR, Fitzgerald NC, Doughty DG, et al. Topical palmitoyl pentapeptide provides improvement in photoaged human facial skin. Int J Cosmet Sci 2005;27:158; with permission.)

that their interaction maintains the antioxidant reservoir within the skin. A combination of 15% ascorbic acid and 1% alpha tocopherol versus vehicle solution were applied to pig skin for 4 days and exposed to irradiation, resulting in a 4-fold antioxidant protection compared with control as well as protected against thymine dimer formation.[35] Ferulic acid, a plant antioxidant, has also been studied for its synergistic effect in combination with vitamin C and E formulations, leading to improved chemical stability and doubled

photoprotection as measured by erythema and sunburn cell formation, as well as a reduction in thymine dimer formation.[36] In a study of 10 participants, an antioxidant mixture composed of vitamin C, ferulic acid, and phloretin versus a vehicle control was applied to human skin, which was then subjected to UV irradiation. Photodamage effects, including sunburn cell formation, thymine dimer formation, matrix metalloproteinase expression, and p53 expression, were all abrogated with the application of the antioxidant

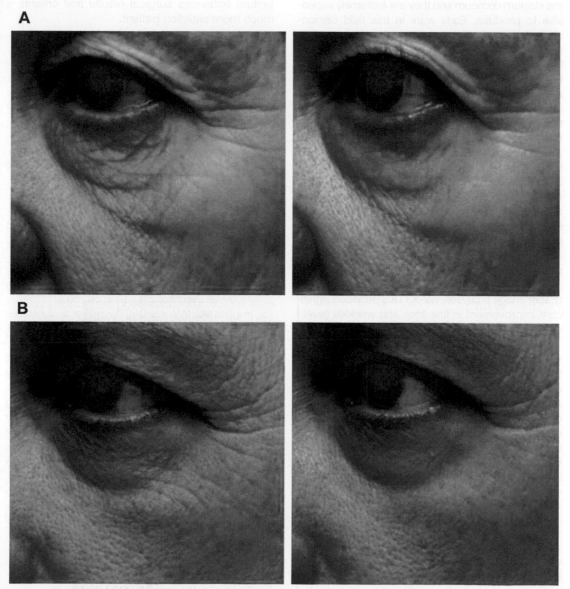

Fig. 6. (*A*) Niacinimide/peptide/retinyl proprionate regimen before and after 8 weeks of topical treatment. (*B*) Tretinoin regimen before and after 8 weeks of treatment. (*From* Fu JJ, Hillebrand GG, Raleigh P, et al. A randomized, controlled, comparative study of the wrinkle reduction benefits of a cosmetic niacinamide/peptide/retinyl propionate product regimen vs a prescription 0.02% tretinoin product regimen. Br J Dermatol 2010;162:651; with permission.)

compound. In addition, UV-related signs of immu-nosuppression, including a reduction in the number of Langerhans cells, was also identified with topical application of antioxidant mixture.[37]

GROWTH FACTORS AND PEPTIDES

Growth factors and peptides represent an emerging field in cosmeceuticals for photoaging. Initially, peptides proved challenging to harness for topical application, because they are highly soluble and fragile compounds, with poor skin penetration through the stratum corneum and they are extremely expensive to produce. Early work in this field demonstrated that mindful selection of proper peptide sequences, as well as conjugation with long chain fatty acids, improves skin penetration and makes these compounds a reality for topical use.[38] There are 3 peptide formulations that have recently garnered interest: palmitoyl-lysine-threonine-threonine-lysine-serine (pal-KTTKS; trade name Matrixyl), acetyl-glutamate-glutamate-methionine-glutamate-arginine-arginine (Ac-EEMQRR; trade name Argireline), and copper glycine-histidine-lysine (Cu-GHK) with pal-KTTKS having the most clinical support to date. Human tissue culture studies have demonstrated that pal-KTTKS stimulates collagen production in a concentration-dependent manner.[39] In a double-blind, placebo-controlled, split-face study of 93 patients, pal-KTTKS or vehicle control was applied for 12 weeks. In both quantitative analysis and expert grader image analyses, pal-KTTKS provided significant improvement in fine lines and wrinkles (level I evidence; **Fig. 5**).[40]

Prior literature recommends a dose range for cosmetic applications of 2 to 8 ppm, which is important to note because the cost of the drug increases expeditiously with increasing dosage.[41] As the greatest body of literature exists in support of the efficacy of retinol-based products, there is merit in comparing potentially less irritating cosmeceutical growth factors with the gold standard of topical retinols. To this end, an 8-week randomized parallel group study of 196 women was conducted in 2009 comparing topical application of a peptide-containing moisturizer (composed of niacinimide, 2 peptide mixtures including pal-KTTKS, and retinyl propionate) versus 0.02% tretinoin. Based on expert grading and image analysis as well as self-assessment questionnaires, the peptide mixture group experienced a significant improvement in wrinkle appearance after 8 weeks compared with tretinoin, with comparable benefits after 24 weeks, and was better tolerated than tretinoin (level II evidence, not blinded; **Fig. 6**).[42] This study shows promise for the efficacy

and tolerability of peptide containing cosmeceuticals; however, further studies are needed to tease out the degree of efficacy related to the peptide component of this multi-ingredient compound.

SUMMARY

In a cosmetic facial plastic surgery practice, photoaging is a concern of most every patient. Understanding appropriate use of skin care can help to prevent and reverse photoaging. Refining skin texture enhances surgical results and creates a much more satisfied patient.

REFERENCES

1. Yaar M, Gilchrest BA. Photoageing: mechanism, prevention and therapy. Br J Dermatol 2007;157: 874–87.
2. Kochevar IE. Molecular and cellular effects of UV radiation relevant to chronic photodamage. In: Gilchrest BA, editor. Photodamage. Cambridge (United Kingdom): Blackwell Science; 1995. p. 51.
3. Hillebrand GG, Miyamoto K, Schnell B, et al. Quantitative evaluation of skin condition in an epidemiological survey of females living in northern versus southern Japan. J Dermatol Sci 2001;27(Suppl 1): S42–52.
4. Diffey BL. The impact of topical photoprotectants intended for daily use on lifetime ultraviolet exposure. J Cosmet Dermatol 2011;10(3):245–50.
5. Hughes MC, Williams GM, Baker P, et al. Sunscreen and prevention of skin aging: a randomized trial. Ann Intern Med 2013;158(11):781–90.
6. Mitchnick MA, Fairhurst D, Pinnell SR. Microfine zinc oxide (Z-cote) as a photostable UVA/UVB sunblock agent. J Am Acad Dermatol 1999;40(1):85–90.
7. Food and Drug Administration, HHS. Labeling and effectiveness testing; sunscreen drug products for over-th-counter human use. Final rule. Fed Regist 2011;76(117):36520–65.
8. Mancebo SA, Hu JY, Wang SQ. Sunscreens a review of health benefits, regulations, and controversies. Dermatol Clin 2014;32(3):427–38.
9. Petkovich M, Brand NJ, Krust A, et al. A human retinoic acid receptor which belongs to the family of nuclear receptors. Nature 1987;33:444–50.
10. Fisher GJ, Datta SC, Talwar HS, et al. Molecular basis of sun-induced premature skin ageing and retinoid antagonism. Nature 1996;379:335–9.
11. Fisher GJ, Voorhees JJ. Molecular mechanisms of retinoid actions in skin. FASEB J 1996;10:1002–13.
12. Kligman AM, Grove GL, Hirose R, et al. Topical tretinoin for photoaged skin. J Am Acad Dermatol 1986;15:836–59.

13. Bhawan J. Short- and long-term histologic effects of topical tretinoin on photodamaged skin. Int J Dermatol 1998;37:286–92.

14. Talwar HS, Griffiths CE, Fisher GJ, et al. Reduced type I and type III procollagens in photodamaged adult human skin. J Invest Dermatol 1995;105:285–90.

15. Griffiths CE, Russman AN, Majmudar G, et al. Restoration of collagen formation in photodamaged human skin by tretinoin (retinoic acid). N Engl J Med 1993;329:530–5.

16. Weiss JS, Ellis CN, Headington JT, et al. Topical tretinoin improves photoaged skin: a double-blind vehicle-controlled study. JAMA 1988;259:527–32.

17. Weinstein GD, Nigra TP, Pochi PE, et al. Topical tretinoin for treatment of photodamaged skin: a multicenter study. Arch Dermatol 1991;127:659–65.

18. Olsen EA, Katz HI, Levine N, et al. Tretinoin emollient cream: a new therapy for photodamaged skin. J Am Acad Dermatol 1992;26:215–24.

19. Kang S, Bergfeld W, Gottlieb AB, et al. Long-term efficacy and safety of tretinoin emollient cream 0.05% in the treatment of photodamaged facial skin: a two-year, randomized, placebo-controlled trial. Am J Clin Dermatol 2005;6:245–53.

20. Bagati E, Guadanhim LR, Enokihara MM, et al. Low-dose oral isotretinoin versus topical retinoic acid for photoaging: a randomized, comparative study. Int J Dermatol 2014;53(1):114–22.

21. Babamiri K, Nassab R. Cosmeceuticals: the evidence behind the retinoids. Aesthet Surg J 2010; 30(1):74–7.

22. Van Scott EJ, Yu RJ. Control of keratinization with alpha hydroxyacids and related compounds. I. Topical treatment of ichthyotic disorders. Arch Dermatol 1974;110(4):586–90.

23. Okano Y, Abe Y, Masaki H, et al. Biological effects of glycolic acid on dermal matrix metabolism medicated by dermal fibroblasts and epidermal keratinocytes. Exp Dermatol 2003;12(Suppl 2):57–63.

24. Ditre CM, Griffin TD, Murphy GF, et al. Effects of alpha-hydroxy acids on photoaged skin: a pilot clinical, histologic, and ultrastructural study. J Am Acad Dermatol 1996;34:187–95.

25. Bernstein EF, Lee J, Brown DB, et al. Glycolic acid treatment increases type I collagen mRNA and hyaluronic acid content of human skin. Dermatol Surg 2001;27(5):429–33.

26. Alster TS, West TB. Effect of topical vitamin C on postoperative carbon dioxide laser resurfacing erythema. Dermatol Surg 1998;24:331–4.

27. Leveque N, Muret P, Mary S, et al. Decrease in skin ascorbic acid concentration with age. Eur J Dermatol 2002;12:XXI–II.

28. Tajima S, Pinnell SR. Ascorbic acid preferentially enhances type I and III collagen gene transcription in human skin fibroblasts. J Dermatol Sci 1996;11: 250–3.

29. Nusgens BV, Humbert P, Rougier A, et al. Topically applied vitamin C enhances the mRNA level of collagens I and III, their processing enzymes and tissue inhibitor of matrix metalloproteinase 1 in the human dermis. J Invest Dermatol 2001;116:853–9.

30. Traikovich SS. Use of topical ascorbic acid and its effects on photodamaged skin topography. Arch Otolaryngol Head Neck Surg 1999;125:1091–8.

31. Fitzpatrick RW, Rostan EF. Double-blind, half-face study comparing topical vitamin C and vehicle for rejuvenation of photodamage. Dermatol Surg 2002; 28:231–6.

32. Humbert PG, Haftek M, Creidi P, et al. Topical ascorbic acid on photoaged skin: clinical, topographical and ultrastructural evaluation: double-blind study versus placebo. Exp Dermatol 2003; 12:237–44.

33. Darr D, Combs S, Dunston S, et al. Topical vitamin C protects porcine skin from ultraviolet radiation-induced damage. Br J Dermatol 1992;127:247–53.

34. Nakamura T, Pinnell SR, Darr D, et al. Vitamin C abrogates the deleterious effects of UVB radiation on cutaneous immunity by a mechanism that does not depend on TNF-alpha. J Invest Dermatol 1997;109: 20–4.

35. Lin JY, Selim MA, Shea CR, et al. UV photoprotection by combination topical antioxidants vitamin and vitamin E. J Am Acad Dermatol 2003;48:866–74.

36. Lin FH, Lin JY, Gupta RD, et al. Ferulic acid stabilizes a solution of vitamins C and E and doubles its photoprotection of skin. J Invest Dermatol 2005; 125:826–32.

37. Oresajo C, Stephens T, Hino PD, et al. Protective effects of a topical antioxidant mixture containing vitamin C, ferulic acid, and phloretin against ultraviolet-induced photodamage in human skin. J Cosmet Dermatol 2008;7:290–7.

38. Lintner K, Peschard O. Biologically active peptides: from a laboratory bench curiosity to a functional skin care product. Int J Cosmet Sci 2000;22:207–18.

39. Jones RR, Vastelletto V, Connon CJ, et al. Collagen stimulating effect of peptide amphiphile C_{16}-KTTS on human fibroblasts. Mol Pharm 2013;10(3):1063–9.

40. Robinson LR, Fitzgerald NC, Doughty DG, et al. Topical palmitoyl pentapeptide provides improvement in photoaged human facial skin. Int J Cosmet Sci 2005;27:155–60.

41. Graf J. Anti-aging skin care ingredient technologies. In: Burgess CM, editor. Cosmetic dermatology. Berlin; Heidelberg (Germany): Springer-Verlag; GmbH & Co KG; 2005. p. 17–28.

42. Fu JJ, Hillebrand GG, Raleigh P, et al. A randomized, controlled, comparative study of the wrinkle reduction benefits of a cosmetic niacinamide/peptide/retinyl propionate product regimen vs a prescription 0.02% tretinoin product regimen. Br J Dermatol 2010;162:647–54.

Evidence-Based Medicine in Laser Medicine for Facial Plastic Surgery

Benjamin C. Marcus, MD*, David Hyman, MD

KEYWORDS

- Skin resurfacing • Ablative laser resurfacing • Broad-band light • Non-invasive skin tightening

KEY POINTS

- Ablative skin resurfacing provides reliable improvement in skin texture.
- Non-surgical skin tightening has moderate evidence for efficacy.
- Light-based therapies are safe and effective for improving sun-damaged skin.

INTRODUCTION

The field of facial laser medicine is at the nexus of multiple medical specialties. Facial plastic surgery, dermatology, and plastic surgery each have significant demand for facial rejuvenation and improvement without surgery. Given this high degree of demand, it should come as no surprise that there is a rapidly enlarging market for new technologies. In a setting in which there are multiple technologies and rapid change, it can be difficult to determine what specific technologies will deliver the results for patients. There is even more confusion for practitioners, as the intense market competition can force manufacturers to make bold claims about their devices in a hope to capture market share.

This is the exact scenario in which evidence-based medicine (EBM) can be most useful. In the setting of rapidly changing technology, tone must make a decision on whether he or she places a premium on being an early adopter of technology or delay purchasing decisions until there is adequate proof that a particular technology is useful. Early adopters will have the obvious advantage of being first and attracting certain types of patients who will want the newest laser technology. Laser devices are a significant capital expenditure; therefore members of the second group who base their purchasing decisions on EBM may be able to avoid deploying capitol into a purchase that becomes obsolete as quickly as it appears.

Another equally critical reason to pursue and utilize EBM in laser medicine is to accurately and effectively communicate expectations with potential patients. Although it may be clear what degree and type of improvement are possible with traditional ablative laser resurfacing, it can be much more difficult to quantify for patients the changes they can expect with newer nonablative technologies. Happy patients are well counseled and have proper expectations set. EBM is a great way to communicate likely outcomes that depart from the traditional and sometimes unsupported claims of manufacturers. In no way should this article dissuade practitioners from utilizing or purchasing devices that they are interested in. Rather the authors hope that this article would serve as an additional reference and help facial cosmetic physicians determine what devices might be right for them.

Disclosure Statement: The authors have no relevant financial disclosures or conflicts of interest.
Section of Facial Plastic Surgery, Division of Otolaryngology, Department of Surgery, University of Wisconsin, Madison, WI, USA
* Corresponding author. 600 Highland Avenue, Madison, WI 53717.
E-mail address: marcus@surgery.wisc.edu

Facial Plast Surg Clin N Am 23 (2015) 297–302
http://dx.doi.org/10.1016/j.fsc.2015.04.003
1064-7406/15/$ – see front matter © 2015 Elsevier Inc. All rights reserved.

NON-INVASIVE TECHNOLOGIES

Nonablative laser devices are among the fastest growing sections of laser medicine. Much of this is, of course, driven by patient demand. Devices in this category include light therapy devices such as Intense Pulsed Light (IPL), Broad Band Light (BBL, Sciton, Palo Alto, California) and a multitude of devices that are designed to improve skin laxity without external wounds or down time. Not surprisingly, each of these devices and their attractive marketing campaigns generate significant patient interest. In this section, the authors will collate the available data and attempt to discern what devices have data to back up their claims.

Intense Pulsed Light and Broad Band Light

IPL was originally approved by the US Food and Drug Administration (FDA) for the treatment of telangiectasia in 1995. It has gone on to have an expanded series of indications and is currently used for treating vascular lesions, pigmented skin lesions, and even hair removal. Multiple generations of devices have been produced and its newest iteration is called BBL. This device has marketing that suggests that regular treatment with BBL can slow or even reverse the aging process. The authors will examine the data to determine what one can safely convey to patients in regards to these devices.

The IPL devices have been clinically successful at reducing solar lentigo and capillaries. When moving beyond the clinical anecdote toward EBM, one needs to have studies that can confirm or deny what is seen clinically. A useful study from 2007 does just that[1] (level 4 evidence). In this study, treatment groups were split into primary capillary (rosacea) or melanosis groups (solar lentigines). Treatments were performed at standard settings (fluence 21 J/cm^2; pulse width 20 ms; spot size 10 × 15 mm^2), and a spectrophotometric analysis of photography was performed (**Fig. 1**). The therapy was particularly effective for rosacea-type skin, with post-treated lesions

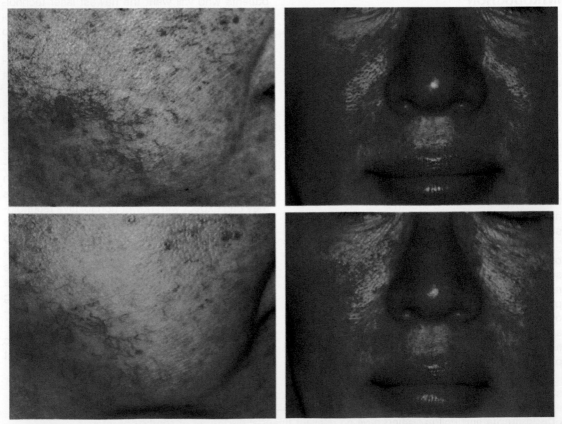

Fig. 1. Effects of intense pulsed light on rosacea lesions. (Left column) Erythematotelangiectatic rosacea (case 1) and (right column) papulopustular rosacea (case 7). Erythema and telangiectasia were remarkably attenuated after 3 treatments in both cases, but some papules and pustules still remained in case 7. Row 1, pretreatment area. Row 2, after treatment. (*From* Kawana S, Ochiai H, Tachihara R. Objective evaluation of the effect of intense pulsed light on rosacea and solar lentigines by spectrophotometric analysis of skin color. Dermatol Surg 2007;33(4):449–54; with permission.)

approaching appearance of normal skin areas (efficacy rate, 91.6%, N = 12). For patients with solar lentigines, skin was also significantly improved after a single treatment (efficacy rate, 66.6%, N = 18). Most therapeutic programs involve more than 1 session of IPL, but this study presents a clear and effective model for evaluating the results of IPL treatment in an objective fashion. Each arm of the study had fewer than 20 patients, but most importantly, this study confirms in a scientific fashion an already known clinical effect.

A much less certain clinical effect is if IPL or BBL treatments improve skin texture in addition to color. A key element for understanding the effects of IPL therapy on skin is to compare and correlate clinical outcomes with changes in underlying histology. In other words, does treatment with IPL cause changes in the actual texture of the skin, and can this be seen at the histologic level? In a study from 2011, El-Domyati and colleagues[2] evaluated patients undergoing IPL and then obtained preauricular skin biopsies (level 4 evidence). These evaluated for histologic changes. They performed quantitative evaluation of collagen types I, III, and VII; newly synthesized collagen; total elastin; and tropoelastin for skin biopsies at baseline, end of treatment, and 3 months after treatment. Although all patients noticed an improvement in the color variegation of their skin, no one reported improvement in fine lines or wrinkles. Although this study was limited by having only 6 patients, it takes a step in the right direction by utilizing objective analysis of skin components known to be associated with regeneration and presumable renewed skin architecture.

The more significant the claim, the more rigorous the proof needs to be to support that claim. Over the last 18 months, the BBL device has been marketed as a device that can slow and even reverse the aging process. A recent pilot study has attempted to elucidate this claim[3] (level 2 evidence). The authors found that skin aging was associated with a significantly altered expression level of 2265 coding and noncoding RNAs. This was studied by looking at gene array expression. Samples that were evaluated after BBL treatments saw changes in 1293 of these gene products. When compared with younger skin controls (N = 5), the treated gene arrays (N = 5) became more similar to their expression level in youthful skin. The genes that underwent an alteration in expression included several known key regulators of organismal and cellular aging. This study is a fine example of the type of research that should be pursued to substantiate claims of device effectiveness. However, further study, including refinement of what genes are affected and how this regulates cellular aging, should be pursued.

Noninvasive Skin Tightening Devices

Achieving tightening of facial and neck skin without surgery is understandably one of the most sought after treatments by patients. There are a multitude of different devices that purport to improve skin tone and correct elastosis. Energy types include infrared, ultrasound, and radiofrequency (RF) ablation, In general, these devices function by sending their selected energy to the deeper layers of the dermis while bypassing the epidermis and creating increases in temperature that result in tightening or wounding of the dermis. The hallmark of each of these treatments is a minimum of any downtime and gradual reversal of elastosis. This particular subset of treatments is seductive for patients. The marketing is slick, and the potential risks seem low. To best advise one's patients, it is critical to utilize EBM and communicate what is known scientifically rather than clinical anecdote or marketing hyperbole.

One of the market leaders in noninvasive skin tightening is Ultherapy (Ulthera, Mesa, Arizona). This device uses highly focused ultrasound to bypass the epidermis and create microwounds in the dermis. These lesions initiate a wound healing response and creation of new collagen and elastin. Certainly there is experimental evidence that demonstrates that the basic scientific premise is there. A study in 2008[4] showed that the experimental ultrasound device could indeed produce microwounds inside the dermis with precise localization (level 4 evidence). The study also confirmed histologic changes consistent with coagulation and initial collagen breakdown. The limitation of this study was that it was performed in samples of human cadaver skin. Obviously this does not allow one to observe if new collagen or elastin production occurs. Although the authors applaud any study that utilizes histologic analysis for evaluating skin changes, this is not enough to make clinical recommendations.

The best modality for determining likely patient outcomes is a true clinical trial. Authors in South Korea recently completed a trial of highly focused ultrasound on the lower eyelids[5] (level 4 evidence). The authors evaluated patient satisfaction with standard analog tools (scale 1–5). More importantly, they obtained objective data by obtaining pretreatment and post-treatment orbital computed tomography (CT) scans. Based on the CT images, the difference between the pre- and postoperative distances from the baseline to the most protruding point of the orbital septum was indeed statistically different for both the right and left eyes. These particular types of objective data are what is required to truly substantiate devices of this nature. What is missing from the study and would be useful for future studies is what happens at 6 months, 12 months, or even several years out from the treatment. In other words, one needs to answer the key patient question: how long does this last?

Ultrasound appears to be most helpful in thin patients and much less so in patients with elevated body mass index (BMI) based on results from a larger lower facial study completed in late 2014[6] (level 2 evidence). This study had over 100 patients and followed them for 3 months. Subjective blinded evaluators were combined with computer CAD-assisted measurements. Ninety-three patients were evaluated. Blinded reviewers observed improvement in skin laxity in 58.1% of patients. Through quantitative assessments, overall improvement in skin laxity was noted in 63.6% of evaluated patients. No change was detected in 54.5% of patients whose BMI exceeded 30 kg/m^2 or in the 12.2% of patients whose BMI was $\leq$30 kg/m^2. Once again, this study provides actual

facts that can be discussed with patients. The key study, which has not yet been performed, is to make the objective measurements at longer intervals out from the primary treatment. This is key to advising patients on treatment decisions. Ultrasound may indeed improve a subset of patients, but 3-month follow up is insufficient to make long-term recommendations.

Another modality that is popular for noninvasive skin tightening is RF ablation. Overall effectiveness of RF ablation has been harder to determine.[7] In a study that compared RF ablation with facelift surgery, the results showed improvements relative to baseline 16% for RF ablation treatment compared with 49% for the surgical face-lift (level 1 evidence). Despite the limited amount of change, patient satisfaction was high.

A recent interesting study compared the histologic effects of highly focused ultrasound and RF ablation[8] (level 4 evidence). They measured neocollagenesis and neoelastogenesis in each layer of the dermis in the area of fraction before and after

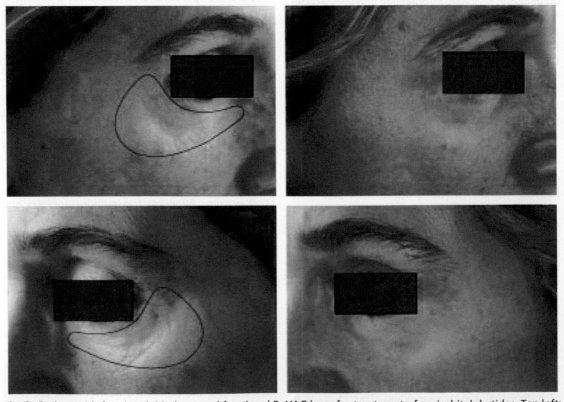

Fig. 2. Patient with fractional CO$_2$ laser and fractional Er:YAG laser for treatment of periorbital rhytides. Top left: preoperative appearance (*black line* demarcates the treatment area). Top right: 3 months postoperatively (CO$_2$). Bottom left: preoperative appearance. Bottom right: 3 months postoperatively (Er:YAG). Marked reduction in rhytides on both sides. (*From* Karsai S, Czarnecka A, Jünger M, et al. Ablative fractional lasers (CO$_2$ and Er:YAG): a randomized controlled double-blind split-face trial of the treatment of periorbital rhytides. Lasers Surg Med 2010;42(2):160–7; with permission.)

treatment. Ultrasound showed the highest level of neocollagenesis and neoelastogenesis in the deep reticular dermis. Overall, ultrasound better affected deep tissues and impacted more isolated regions. RF ablation also affected deep tissues, but appeared to alter more diffuse regions. This histologic analysis may shed light on why the ultrasound devices appear to have more effect on skin tightening.

ABLATIVE TECHNOLOGIES

Ablative technologies are much less controversial. In general, significant skin ablation results in predictable changes in skin texture. Split face studies are very useful. This allows investigators to compare the effectiveness with an internal control. A study from 2010 evaluated carbon dioxide (CO_2) versus Er:YAG modalities[9] (level 1 evidence). This study had 28 patients. Patients were randomized to a single treatment on each side of the periorbital region, one with a fractional CO^2 laser, and one with a fractional Er:YAG laser. The evaluation included the profilometric measurement of wrinkle depth, the Fitzpatrick wrinkle score. Both lasers showed a roughly equivalent effect (**Fig. 2**). Wrinkle depth and Fitzpatrick score were reduced by approximately 20% and 10%, respectively, with no statistical difference between lasers. Other conclusions were that multiple sessions are required to achieve the ideal effect. Although most fractional lasers demonstrate a degree of effectiveness,[10,11] what is more exciting is some of the effects that have been recently demonstrated in early wound healing with fractional ablative therapy.

One of the more recent and exciting uses for fractional laser therapy is modulation of healing scars. Practitioners have been utilizing a mixture of IPL and fractionated ablative resurfacing to improve outcomes of immature scars. Recently published,[12] a prospective randomized, comparative split-scar study was conducted on 20 subjects (Level II Evidence). These were patients who underwent Mohs surgery. Eligible subjects were those with a linear scar of 4 cm or greater. At suture removal (between 7–10 days) CO2 fractional laser was performed. Scars were re-evaluated 12 weeks later using the Vancouver scar scale (VSS) and patient completed visual analog scale (VAS). While the VSS improvement did not reach significance, the VAS rating was significantly improved for treated scar (**Fig. 3**).

An important head-to-head study comparing fractional ablative resurfacing with full-field ablative resurfacing was also recently completed.[13] Clinical improvement was not significantly different between the 2 systems; however,

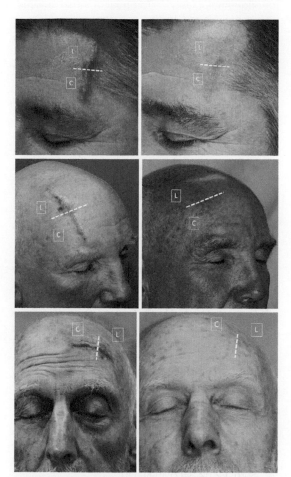

Fig. 3. Three patients with split-scar early fractional laser treatment for surgical scar. Left: 1 week postoperative appearance. Right: 12 weeks postoperative appearance (L $\frac{1}{4}$ laser treated half, C $\frac{1}{4}$ control). (*From* Sobanko JF, Vachiramon V, Rattanaumpawan P, et al. Early postoperative single treatment ablative fractional lasing of Mohs micrographic surgery facial scars: a split-scar, evaluator-blinded study. J Lasers Surg Med 2015;47(1):1–5; with permission.)

full-field ablation was better at reducing scar hardness, whereas fractional laser was superior for lightening color. These data suggest that combined treatment may be useful to achieve ideal results. This study is well constructed, as it has internal controls and is randomized and prospective. As with all pilot studies, these findings are interesting and useful, but better powered studies will be required to truly prove efficacy.

Lasers have become a crucial tool for facial cosmetic surgeons. With the continued refining of traditional ablative technologies and the development of newer nonablative technologies, there exists greater variability in the devices that may be used. EBM is the best resource for both guiding practitioners in making new technology purchases and for counseling patients in treatment options and outcome expectations. This article is a survey of some of the best EBM for facial cosmetic surgeons available at this time regarding laser technologies.

REFERENCES

1. Kawana S, Ochiai H, Tachihara R. Objective evaluation of the effect of intense pulsed light on rosacea and solar lentigines by spectrophotometric analysis of skin color. Dermatol Surg 2007;33(4):449–54.
2. El-Domyati M, El-Ammawi TS, Moawad O, et al. Intense pulsed light photorejuvenation: a histological and immunohistochemical evaluation. J Drugs Dermatol 2011;10(11):1246–52.
3. Chang AL, Bitter PH Jr, Qu K, et al. Rejuvenation of gene expression pattern of aged human skin by broadband light treatment: a pilot study. J Invest Dermatol 2013;133(2):394–402.
4. Laubach HJ, Makin IR, Barthe PG, et al. Intense focused ultrasound: evaluation of a new treatment modality for precise microcoagulation within the skin. Dermatol Surg 2008;34(5):727–34.
5. Pak CS, Lee YK, Jeong JH, et al. Safety and efficacy of ulthera in the rejuvenation of aging lower eyelids: a pivotal clinical trial. Aesthetic Plast Surg 2014; 38(5):861–8.
6. Oni G, Hoxworth R, Teotia S, et al. Evaluation of a microfocused ultrasound system for improving skin laxity and tightening in the lower face. Aesthet Surg J 2014;34(7):1099–110.
7. Alexiades-Armenakas M, Rosenberg D, Renton B, et al. Blinded, randomized, quantitative grading comparison of minimally invasive, fractional radiofrequency and surgical face-lift to treat skin laxity. Arch Dermatol 2010;146(4):396–405.
8. Suh DH, Choi JH, Lee SJ, et al. Comparative histometric analysis of the effects of high intensity focused ultrasound (HIFU) and radiofrequency (RF) on skin. J Cosmet Laser Ther 2015;1–22.
9. Karsai S, Czarnecka A, Jünger M, et al. Ablative fractional lasers (CO(2) and Er:YAG): a randomized controlled double-blind split-face trial of the treatment of peri-orbital rhytides. Lasers Surg Med 2010;42(2):160–7.
10. Kohl E, Meierhöfer J, Koller M, et al. Fractional carbon dioxide laser resurfacing of rhytides and photoaged skin—a prospective clinical study on patient expectation and satisfaction. Lasers Surg Med 2015;47(2):111–9.
11. Kauvar AN. Fractional nonablative laser resurfacing: is there a skin tightening effect? Dermatol Surg 2014;40(Suppl 12):S157–63.
12. Sobanko JF, Vachiramon V, Rattanaumpawan P, et al. Early postoperative single treatment ablative fractional lasing of Mohs micrographic surgery facial scars: a split-scar, evaluator-blinded study. Lasers Surg Med 2015;47(1):1–5.
13. Ortiz AE, Goldman MP, Fitzpatrick RE. Ablative CO2 lasers for skin tightening: traditional versus fractional. Dermatol Surg 2014;40:S147–51.

Evidence-Based Medicine
Rhinoplasty

Matthew K. Lee, MD[a], Sam P. Most, MD[b],*

KEYWORDS

- Evidence based medicine • Functional rhinoplasty • Nasal valve stenosis • Cosmetic rhinoplasty
- Aesthetic rhinoplasty • Systematic reviews

KEY POINTS

- Outcomes in rhinoplasty can be assessed by subjective, objective, and clinician-reported measures.
- Use of validated measures ensures reliability and consistency in outcomes reporting.
- Although most studies demonstrate near-universal support for the efficacy of functional and aesthetic rhinoplasty techniques, future studies should emphasize use of validated outcome measures when reporting data.
- Although level 1 evidence studies are currently rare in rhinoplasty literature, evidence-based medicine can be applied to rhinoplasty based on the wealth of data available from case reports, case series, cohort studies, experiments without controls, statements of expert opinion, and basic science research.

INTRODUCTION

The practice of evidence-based medicine has become increasingly prominent in the climate of modern day health care. The current pace of technologic innovation has led to the rapid development of novel medical therapies, each necessitating proof of efficacy, safety, and utility. Increasingly, physicians have come to consider evidence-based decision-making as the standard of care, a development that has been paralleled by matching expectations from patients. Far from replacing the traditional teachings of medicine, evidence-based medicine requires the integration of clinical experience and expertise in conjunction with the best available evidence and individual patient values and preferences.[1]

The Oxford Center for Evidence-Base Medicine has developed one of the most widely recognized classifications systems for critically appraising the strength of clinical evidence. At the upper echelon of this 5-tiered schema are systematic reviews of randomized controlled trials (level 1 evidence), followed by comparison cohort studies (level 2), case-control studies (level 3 evidence), case series (level 4), and expert opinion and bench research (level 5). A common mistake is the assumption that higher levels of evidence invariably represent better evidence. This is particularly relevant to the surgical specialties because level 1 evidence data are rare given the inherent ethical concerns in randomizing patients into a placebo treatment (ie, sham surgery) group. Fortunately, although the prevalence of level 1 evidence data may be relatively limited in facial plastic and reconstructive surgery, advancement of knowledge may occur through alternative study designs, including cohort

Financial Disclosures: None.

[a] Division of Facial Plastic and Reconstructive Surgery, Stanford University School of Medicine, 801 Welch Road, Stanford, CA 94305, USA; [b] Division of Facial Plastic and Reconstructive Surgery, Department of Otolaryngology – Head and Neck Surgery, Stanford University School of Medicine, 801 Welch Road, Stanford, CA 94305, USA

* Corresponding author.

E-mail address: smost@ohns.stanford.edu

Facial Plast Surg Clin N Am 23 (2015) 303–312

http://dx.doi.org/10.1016/j.fsc.2015.04.004

1064-7406/15/$ – see front matter © 2015 Elsevier Inc. All rights reserved.

studies, experiments without controls, uncontested expert opinion, or basic scientific research.[1] These types of studies have helped facial plastic surgeons navigate a world in which evidence-based medicine is not considered a luxury but, instead, the standard of care.

The term rhinoplasty when used broadly refers to surgery of the nose that is undertaken either to improve aesthetics, nasal function, or both. When the primary goal of surgery is to improve the appearance of the nose, this is typically specified as aesthetic or cosmetic rhinoplasty. When the primary goal of surgery is to improve nasal function by repair of an anatomic source of obstruction, it is referred to as functional rhinoplasty or nasal valve repair, with these terms often used interchangeably. The goal of this article is to provide a brief summary of current outcomes data regarding functional and aesthetic rhinoplasty surgery to help facilitate evidence-based clinical decision-making.

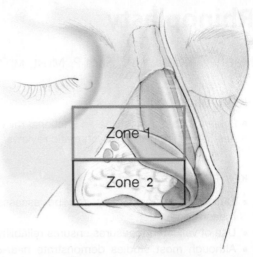

Fig. 1. Green box, Zone 1, corresponds to the scroll region and inferior upper lateral cartilage. Blue box, Zone 2, akin to the traditionally described external nasal valve.

FUNCTIONAL RHINOPLASTY
Outcome Evaluation in Functional Rhinoplasty

Assessing clinical outcomes following functional rhinoplasty surgery has remained a highly controversial topic. It has long been recognized that significant incongruities can exist between a patient's self-reported severity of nasal obstruction and objective measurements of nasal valve function.[2] The nasal valve defines the area of the nasal passages with the smallest cross-sectional area and, therefore, the highest resistance to airflow. Traditionally, it is taught that the nasal valve has 2 components, internal and external, that can be involved with nasal valve compromise and nasal obstruction. The internal nasal valve is defined by the caudal edge of the upper lateral cartilages, the septum, and the anterior inferior turbinate. The angle formed between the upper lateral cartilage and the dorsal septum is critical for maintaining patency of the internal nasal valve, with the normative range being between 10° to 15°. The external nasal valve is defined by the nasal ala, caudal septum, the caudal aspect of the lower lateral cartilages, and nasal sill.[3]

More recent nomenclature has taken into account the dynamic nature of nasal valve obstruction, using the term lateral wall insufficiency (LWI) to refer to the inspiratory collapse of the lateral wall.[4] LWI can be further divided into 2 zones (Fig. 1). Zone 1 is located more cephalad and corresponds to the scroll region and inferior upper lateral cartilage. Zone 2 is akin to the traditionally described external valve. It is located caudal to Zone 1 and corresponds to the skin and soft tissues of the nasal ala.

Generally, assessment of treatment efficacy and outcomes in functional rhinoplasty can be divided into 3 categories: objective measures of nasal function, patient-reported measures, and clinician-derived measures.

Objective anatomic measures
Objective measures can be further subcategorized as either anatomic (measuring structural dimensions) or physiologic (measuring functional or biological parameters).[2] There is much debate regarding the value of objective measures in the assessment of nasal valve compromise and clinical nasal obstruction and, as such, these are used primarily for research purposes instead of for clinical decision-making.

Objective anatomic measures include acoustic rhinometry and radiographic studies assessing nasal cavity dimensions and geometry. Acoustic rhinometry is a diagnostic measure that uses acoustic reflections to calculate nasal airway cross-sectional area as a function of longitudinal distance along the nasal passageway. Nasal passage volumes can then be calculated from contiguous cross-sectional values. This allows for assessment of the dimension of the nasal airway at specific points along the nasal passage.[5] Although its clinical applications are still debated, acoustic rhinometry has seen widespread adoption in clinical research with more than 500 studies published since the late 1980s.[6] Importantly, acoustic rhinometry is a static measurement of nasal dimensions and, therefore, measurements may vary depending on the degree of current nasal congestion. It is, therefore, important to obtain measurements both before and after topical decongestion in order to distinguish between mucosal hypertrophy and true structural deformity.[6]

High-resolution computed tomography (CT) can also be used to directly obtain anatomic measurements of the nasal dimensions instead of the indirect methods used by acoustic rhinometry. In a level 4 case series validating high-resolution CT against acoustic rhinometry, cross-sectional areas and nasal cavity volumes from each method showed significant correlation.[7] Like acoustic rhinometry, it is a static measurement of nasal dimensions and is subject to physiologic variations in nasal mucosal congestion. One additional benefit of radiographic imaging studies is that the angle of the internal nasal valve can be measured. Because the angle of the internal nasal valve is known to play a critical role in nasal valve compromise, this provides additional diagnostic information that can be used in surgical decision making.[8]

Objective physiologic measures

Physiologic measures include rhinomanometry and measurements of peak nasal inspiratory flow. Rhinomanometry is a dynamic diagnostic tool that measures transnasal pressure and nasal volume airflow to calculate nasal airway resistance during nasal inspiration. Generally, rhinomanometry can be differentiated into active and passive methods, with each of these being subdivided further into anterior and posterior techniques.[9] In practice, the active anterior method is the most commonly used because it is the most physiologic technique.[10] In the active anterior technique, the patient actively breathes through one nasal cavity while the transnasal pressure (the difference in pressure from the naris to the nasopharynx) is measured with a pressure probe in the contralateral nostril.[6]

Nasal peak inspiratory flow is another noninvasive physiologic measure that measures the maximum airflow that the subject is able to produce during forced nasal inspiration. It is a reliable method of measuring nasal patency and has been validated against rhinomanometry as well as other objective measures of nasal patency.[2] One significant drawback of this measure is that it includes several potentially confounding factors, including effort dependence and pulmonary function.[11]

Patient-reported outcome measures

In contrast to objective measures, patient-reported outcome measures focus on evaluating the subjective experience of the patient and their self-reported assessment of the efficacy of a given treatment. These measures focus on quality-of-life

(QOL) issues and provide a quantitative assessment of otherwise subjective results.[12] Because the primary goal of functional rhinoplasty surgery is to improve nasal obstructive symptoms, QOL measures have been commonly used to evaluate efficacy of surgery. Disease-specific measures are most useful for this because the health status changes from nasal surgery may be too subtle to be appreciated by global instruments.[13] The visual analog scale (VAS) has been one of the most commonly used disease-specific patient-reported tools for assessing nasal function. Patients indicate the severity of nasal obstruction on a linear scale ranging from no obstruction to complete obstruction.[8] More recently, the Nasal Obstruction Symptom Evaluation (NOSE) scale has come into widespread use. Although numerous other scales had been previously described, including the Chronic Sinusitis Survey and the Sino-Nasal Outcome Tool, the NOSE scale is a disease-specific QOL measure that specifically targets issues related to nasal obstruction instead of inflammatory disease. The NOSE scale has been validated as a reliable and responsive measure of QOL issues related to nasal obstruction.[13] The importance of using a validated QOL scale cannot be understated because this allows for consistency in reporting of outcomes.

Clinician-derived measures

Clinician-derived measures are standardized grading scales used after surgery to assess outcomes based on quantifiable physical examination or clinical findings as assessed by the clinician. These are potentially powerful outcome measures that are currently infrequently used. A recently described methodology for description of LWI has been adopted at the authors' institution and several others. In this system, each zone of the lateral wall is individually evaluated for collapse and rated 0 to 3. This measure of LWI has been validated and its use in reporting outcomes of nasal procedures is burgeoning.[14,15] Another recent level 2c study described a clinician-derived measure involving a rating of the size of the anterior inferior turbinates. In this grading scale, inferior turbinate was graded on a scale of 1 to 4 based on the space occupied by the anterior aspect of the inferior turbinate relative to the total space available at the same anteroposterior location in the nasal cavity. Grade 1 inferior turbinate occupies 0% to 25% of the total airway space, grade 2 occupies 26% to 50%, and so forth.[16]

Recently, a severity classification system has been developed to provide a clinical context to patient-reported NOSE scores. NOSE scores were obtained from 345 patients with and without nasal obstructive symptoms. Using receiver operating characteristic curve analysis, NOSE scores were categorized as being mild (range 5–25), moderate (range 30–50), severe (range 55–75), or extreme (range 80–100). This allowed the addition of a clinician-derived report of outcomes to provide context to the subjective patient-reported NOSE scores.[17]

Discordance of objective and subjective outcome measures

One of the most significant criticisms of objective measures of nasal patency and airflow as an indicator of treatment success is that there seems to be a poor correlation between these objective findings and patient-reported obstructive symptoms. Interestingly, nasal sensation of airflow seems to play a critical, though not yet fully understood, role in subjective nasal obstruction.

In one of the most comprehensive studies to date addressing this topic, Lam and colleagues[2] performed a prospective cross-sectional study of 290 subjects evaluating nasal dimensions and function via acoustic rhinometry and nasal peak inspiratory flow, correlating these findings with a subjective measure of nasal obstruction (VAS). Their investigation demonstrated no significant correlation between any of the anatomic, physiologic, and subjective categories of nasal measures (level 4 evidence). In a contrasting level 4 study, Kjaergaard and colleagues[5] compared acoustic rhinometry and nasal peak inspiratory flow results with VAS scores in 2523 subjects. Their investigation yielded findings disparate to the Lam and colleagues[2] study, with highly significant associations demonstrated between the subjective sensation of nasal obstruction and corresponding measures for nasal cavity volume, area, and airflow. In a recent systematic review of 21 studies published on this topic, equivocal data were demonstrated (level 2 evidence). There seemed to be greater correlation between objective and subjective measures when symptomatic nasal obstruction was present. In the absence of nasal symptoms, however, correlation between subjective and objective measures was poor. Clearly, the data are currently inconclusive regarding the clinical value of objective measures. Because many factors may play a role in the subjective sensation of nasal obstruction, it is likely that no single objective test, albeit qualitatively and technically reliable, will reproducibly correlate with this perception.[6]

AESTHETIC RHINOPLASTY
Patient-Reported Outcome Measures

In perhaps no other field is patient satisfaction a more important measure of success than in cosmetic surgery. Although much retrospective and observational data regarding rhinoplasty techniques have been published, most of these studies report outcomes using nonvalidated, qualitative assessments of patient and/or surgeon satisfaction with results. Interestingly, there are few validated, quantitative outcomes studies in facial plastic and reconstructive surgery despite that patient satisfaction is the primary goal.[18] As with the assessment of nasal obstruction in functional rhinoplasty, validated QOL measures are critical for quantitative assessment of outcomes following aesthetic surgery.

Similar to the NOSE scale, the Rhinoplasty Outcomes Evaluation (ROE) was initially developed as a specific QOL measure of patient satisfaction following aesthetic rhinoplasty surgery.[18] The validity and reliability of the ROE scale has been subsequently confirmed in a multicenter study, providing one of the first validated, quantitative measures for patient-reported outcomes following aesthetic rhinoplasty.[19] Interestingly, to date, these validated QOL scales (NOSE and ROE) have tended to segregate the aesthetic and functional components of outcome and patient satisfaction. This is a somewhat artificial distinction because nasal form and function are closely associated. For instance, functional correction of nasal valve compromise and simultaneously causing a new aesthetic complaint will most often result in a decrement in overall patient satisfaction. In the future, a comprehensive, disease-specific QOL instrument may be helpful in evaluating patient satisfaction with both form and function of the nose.

Objective Measures

Much has been published on the topic of aesthetic facial analysis and nasal geometry, including normative data and the ideal ranges for a variety of nasal and facial measures. Numerous level 4 and 5 studies have investigated the role of specific rhinoplasty techniques, such as lateral crural repositioning, lateral crural steal, tongue-in-groove sutures, and dorsal reduction on postoperative nasal geometry.[20–22] However, little is understood regarding the correlation between these facial measurements, their relationship to well-described normative ranges, and the subjective assessment of facial beauty.

In an attempt to better understand this relationship, Devcic and colleagues[23] published their investigation into the correlation between 6 methods of measuring nasal tip projection (the Goode, Simons, Baum, Powell, and Crumley methods) with subjective assessment of facial attractiveness in 300 synthetic lateral facial images. Interestingly, they found no significant correlation between any of these ratios and subjective facial attractiveness (level 5 evidence). As with functional rhinoplasty, there does seem to be an incongruity between objective measurements and subjective assessment of outcomes. Similarly, it may be that no individual measurement or proportion can be significantly correlated to the global perception of facial beauty. Nevertheless, these objective measures are important to preoperatively and intraoperatively understanding how various techniques can achieve specific alterations in nasal appearance or measurements.

SURGICAL TECHNIQUES

Nasal obstruction as a consequence of anatomic deformity of the nasal passageways most commonly arises from one or more of 4 areas: septum, inferior turbinates, internal nasal valve, and lateral nasal wall. The terms functional rhinoplasty or nasal valve repair specifically refer to a variety of procedures undertaken to improve nasal obstruction by addressing the anatomic structures that comprise the internal and/or external nasal valves. A treatment algorithm is summarized in **Fig. 2**.

These procedures can be performed individually but are most commonly used in conjunction with surgery of the septum and inferior turbinates. As such, outcomes data for these procedures are reviewed in addition to nasal valve surgery.

Septum

Treatment of the deviated nasal septum by submucous resection with preservation of an intact dorsal and caudal strut (L-strut) was first described by Killian[24] as a means to correct nasal airway obstruction without compromise of the structural integrity of the nose (level 5 evidence). A common maxim of septoplasty surgery is the preservation of a minimum of height of the remnant L-strut at 10 to 15 mm in order to preserve tip projection and prevent saddle nose deformity.[25] However, mechanical testing to assess the validity of this statement was lacking until recent years. Mau and colleagues[25] described their investigation using finite element modeling of maximal tensile stress at the bony cartilaginous junction as a function of L-strut design. Interestingly, their data demonstrated that decreasing the height of the L-strut in half from 15 to 7.5 mm more than doubled the maximal stress at the bony cartilaginous junction. This provided first empiric data supporting the notion that maintenance of an adequate height of the L-strut provides significant additional structural integrity to the nasal skeleton.

Since its description, numerous studies have demonstrated the efficacy of L-strut septoplasty surgery in relief of nasal obstructive symptoms. However, most of these studies used either nonvalidated survey instruments or instruments that were not validated specifically for the assessment of nasal obstruction.[13] In their 2004 publication (level 4 evidence), Stewart and colleagues[26] described the efficacy of septoplasty surgery in a prospective, multicenter study using a validated instrument. In 59 subjects, nasal septoplasty was shown to produce significant improvement in quality of life and nasal obstructive symptoms as measured by the NOSE scale. This provided validated data supporting the efficacy of septoplasty surgery for relief of nasal obstructive symptoms.

One caveat is that traditional septoplasty with preservation of an intact L-strut can preclude complete correction of septal deviation if it involves the caudal aspect of the septal cartilage. Many different techniques for correction of caudal septal deviations have been described. These can be generally categorized into 2 types: in situ septoplasty techniques (including septal repositioning,[27] scoring and morselization,[28] suture techniques,[29] and septal batten graft)[30,31] and extracorporeal septoplasty techniques.[32,33] Generally, in situ septoplasty is reserved for less severe caudal deviations, whereas extracorporeal septoplasty is used in severe deviations or in deviations that persist after in situ techniques. Supporting this notion, Lee and Jang[34] performed a retrospective review comparing these 2 techniques in 169 subjects with caudal septal deviation and found that, although both could be performed with similar aesthetic outcomes, subjects who underwent extracorporeal septoplasty achieved superior functional results and were less likely to suffer from persistent or unresolved nasal obstruction (level 3 evidence).

As with traditional L-strut septoplasty, the efficacy of extracorporeal septoplasty techniques for caudal septal deviations has been supported using validated QOL instruments. In 2006, Most[33] described his experience using a modified extracorporeal septoplasty technique (termed anterior septal reconstruction) for caudal septal deviations. All 12 consecutive subjects had significant improvement in their NOSE scores with an average follow-up of 5.4 months (level 4 evidence). This has been expanded on in a more recent publication reporting outcomes in 77 subjects who underwent anterior septal reconstruction. NOSE and VAS scores were found to be significantly reduced both in the early (<3 months) and late (>3 months) postoperative periods, demonstrating that anterior septal reconstruction represents a powerful

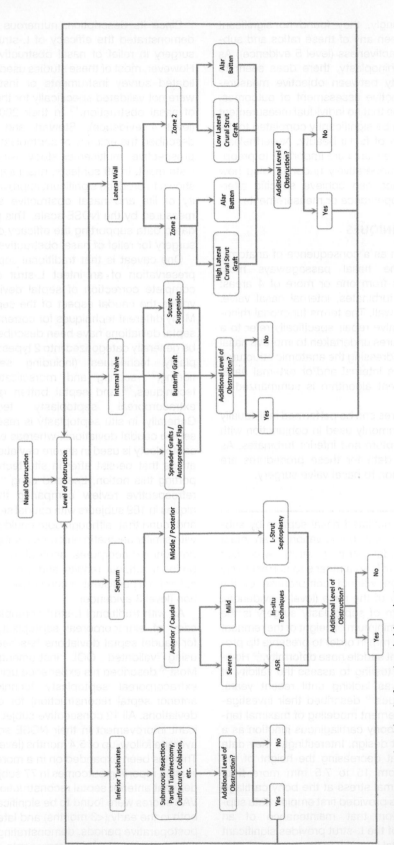

Fig. 2. Treatment algorithm in functional rhinoplasty.

method for correction of nasal valve stenosis resulting from severe anterocaudal septal deviations (level 4 evidence).[35]

Inferior Turbinates

The anterior portion of the inferior turbinate can contribute to obstruction at the level of the internal nasal valve. Accordingly, turbinate reduction procedures are often performed as a component of functional rhinoplasty surgery. Numerous techniques for turbinate reduction have been described in level 4 and level 5 studies, with commonly used methods including partial turbinectomy,[36] submucous resection,[37,38] microdebrider reduction,[39] turbinate outfracture,[40] radiofrequency ablation,[41,42] laser ablation,[43] ultrasound,[44] and submucous coblation.[39]

A comprehensive review of turbinate reduction outcomes was described by Batra and colleagues[45] in 2009. Of the 96 articles that met inclusion criteria, 1 study represented level 1 evidence, 2 studies represented level 2 evidence, 75 studies represented level 4 evidence, and 18 studies represented level 5 evidence. Importantly, only 10 of these studies used validated QOL instruments, including the VAS, NOSE scale, Rhinosinusitis Symptom Inventory, and Likert scale. In studies that used patient-reported outcome measures, subjective symptom improvement was reported in greater than 50% of subjects in 93 of 96 (96.9%) studies. In studies that used objective measures, 14 of 14 acoustic rhinometry studies and 10 of 12 rhinomanometry studies reported improvement in nasal airflow or nasal resistance. Regardless of the technique used, almost all of the data showed significant benefit from surgery, using both objective and subjective measures.

Internal Nasal Valve

As previously described, the term functional rhinoplasty or nasal valve repair does not refer to a single unified procedure but, instead, a collection of various techniques used to correct internal nasal valve compromise. As such, it is difficult to assess the efficacy of any individual technique (eg, spreader grafts, batten grafts) in the correction of nasal valve stenosis because these are almost universally used in conjunction with other related procedures such as septoplasty and turbinate reduction. When looking at the efficacy of functional rhinoplasty as a whole, the current data overwhelmingly demonstrate excellent outcomes regardless of technique used.[46]

In their 2008 article, Rhee and colleagues[47] systematically reviewed the existing outcomes data on functional rhinoplasty techniques during the past

25 years. Of the 44 studies identified, only 2 were categorized as level 2b evidence in which outcomes from different surgical techniques were directly compared. In one of these level 2b studies, septal batten grafts were compared with septal replacement surgery for the treatment of caudal septal deviations, with no statistical difference in obstructive symptoms demonstrated between the 2 treatment groups.[48] The second study with level 2b evidence compared septoplasty alone to nasal valve repair, demonstrating significantly lower postoperative airflow resistance as measured by rhinomanometry in the valvular repair treatment group but not in the septoplasty treatment group.[49] The remaining 44 studies were classified as level 4 evidence. Regardless of the specific techniques applied in each study, there was nearly universal support of the efficacy of functional rhinoplasty with effectiveness ranging from 65% to 100% and no studies showing functional rhinoplasty to be ineffective in the relief of nasal obstruction.[47]

Notably, almost all of these studies did not use validated QOL measurements and only 6 of the 42 studies used validated instruments, including the NOSE scale, Likert satisfaction scale, Epworth Sleepiness Scale, Glasgow Benefit Inventory (GBI), and Nasal Symptom Questionnaire (NSQ). Furthermore, only 3 of these studies used a disease-specific QOL instrument, the NOSE scale. Twelve studies used objective outcome measures, with the most common being rhinomanometry, and one study used nasal plethysmography and measurement of the internal nasal valve. The 3 studies that used a validated, disease-specific QOL instrument were all published within the last 10 years, portending a growing emphasis on the use of validated subjective measures of patient outcome.[47]

Lateral Wall

Traditionally, the nasal valve has been divided into an internal portion and an external potion. Whereas obstruction at the level of the internal nasal valve can be static or dynamic, external valve compromise almost universally refers to a dynamic process occurring with inspiration. As previously described, the term LWI has recently come into use to refer to all dynamic processes of the lateral nasal wall.[4]

Numerous techniques to correct LWI have been described in level 4 and level 5 studies, including alar batten grafts,[50] lateral crural strut grafts,[51] and alar suspension sutures,[52–54] each with specific advantages and disadvantages. As previously described by Rhee and colleagues[47], most these functional rhinoplasty techniques have been described as high efficacious in the relief of the nasal obstruction symptoms. However, few studies have evaluated the efficacy of these techniques as it specifically pertains to treatment of LWI.

To facilitate consistency in communication, a grading scale for LWI has been developed. This grading scale was validated in a recent study in which representative endoscopic videos depicting varied degrees of lateral nasal wall insufficiency were collated into a 30-clip video (15 clips in duplicate). These video clips were then rated by 5 reviewers independently, with very strong interrater and intrarater reliability demonstrated.[14]

This grading scale for LWI has been recently used to assess the efficacy of a novel radiofrequency treatment of the lateral nasal wall. Representing one of the few studies in the facial plastic surgery literature with level 1 evidence data, Weissman and Most[15] have recently described their prospective randomized trial comparing bone-anchored suture technique (BAST) to radiofrequency thermotherapy (RF) for LWI. Significant improvements in subjective NOSE and VAS scores were seen at the 1, 3, 6, and 12 months when compared with preoperative scores for both the RF and BAST treatment arms. Using the aforementioned clinician-derived score of LWI, significant improvement was seen in subjects in the RF group at 1, 6, and 12 months, whereas the BAST group only showed significant improvement at 1 month. Comparison of RF and BAST revealed significant improvement in the RF group over the BAST group at 12 months. Going forward, quantitative assessment of LWI using this validated grading scale would provide a consistent and reliable measure of outcomes following surgery.

SUMMARY

The growth of evidence-based medicine has changed the landscape of facial plastic and reconstructive surgery, for both physicians and for patients. Although level 1 evidence studies are currently rare in this field, a wealth of data from case reports, case series, cohort studies, experiments without controls, statements of expert opinion, and basic science research is available to help facial plastic surgeons use the best available research to complement their clinical decision making. A summary of the current data regarding functional and aesthetic rhinoplasty surgery has been provided.

REFERENCES

1. Rhee JS, Daramola OO. No need to fear evidence-based medicine. Arch Facial Plast Surg 2012; 14(2):89–92.

2. Lam DJ, James KT, Weaver EM. Comparison of anatomic, physiological, and subjective measures of the nasal airway. Am J Rhinol 2006; 20(5):463–70.

3. Rhee JS, Weaver EM, Park SS, et al. Clinical consensus statement: diagnosis and management of nasal valve compromise. Otolaryngol Head Neck Surg 2010;143(1):48–59.

4. Most SP. Trends in functional rhinoplasty. Arch Facial Plast Surg 2008;10(6):410–3.

5. Kjaergaard T, Cvancarova M, Steinsvåg SK. Does nasal obstruction mean that the nose is obstructed? Laryngoscope 2008;118(8):1476–81.

6. André RF, Vuyk HD, Ahmed A, et al. Correlation between subjective and objective evaluation of the nasal airway. A systematic review of the highest level of evidence. Clin Otolaryngol 2009;34(6):518–25.

7. Dastidar P, Numminen J, Heinonen T, et al. Nasal airway volumetric measurement using segmented HRCT images and acoustic rhinometry. Am J Rhinol 1999;13:97–103.

8. Cannon DE, Rhee JS. Evidence-based practice: functional rhinoplasty. Otolaryngol Clin North Am 2012;45(5):1033–43.

9. Naito K, Iwata S. Current advances in rhinomanometry. Eur Arch Otorhinolaryngol 1997;254(7):309–12.

10. Clement PA, Halewyck S, Gordts F, et al. Critical evaluation of different objective techniques of nasal airway assessment: a clinical review. Eur Arch Otorhinolaryngol 2014;271(10):2617–25.

11. Angelos PC, Been MJ, Toriumi DM. Contemporary review of rhinoplasty. Arch Facial Plast Surg 2012; 14(4):238–47.

12. Biggs T, Fraser L, Ward M, et al. Patient reported outcome measures in septorhinoplasty surgery. Ann R Coll Surg Engl 2015;97(1):63–5.

13. Stewart MG, Witsell DL, Smith TL, et al. Development and validation of the nasal obstruction symptom evaluation (NOSE) scale. Otolaryngol Head Neck Surg 2004;130(2):157–63.

14. Tsao GJ, Fijalkowski N, Most SP. Validation of a grading system for lateral nasal wall insufficiency. Allergy Rhinol (Providence) 2013;4(2):e66–8.

15. Weissman JD, Most SP. Radiofrequency thermotherapy vs bone-anchored suspension for treatment of lateral nasal wall insufficiency: a randomized clinical trial. JAMA Facial Plast Surg 2015;17:84–9.

16. Camacho M, Zaghi S, Certal V, et al. Inferior turbinate classification system, grades 1 to 4: development and validation study. Laryngoscope 2015; 125(2):296–302.

17. Lipan MJ, Most SP. Development of a severity classification system for subjective nasal obstruction. JAMA Facial Plast Surg 2013;15(5):358–61.

18. Alsarraf R. Outcomes research in facial plastic surgery: a review and new directions. Aesthetic Plast Surg 2000;24(3):192–7.

19. Alsarraf R, Larrabee WF Jr, Anderson S, et al. Measuring cosmetic facial plastic surgery outcomes: a pilot study. Arch Facial Plast Surg 2001; 3(3):198–201.

20. Datema FR, Lohuis PJ. Tongue-in-groove setback of the medial crura to control nasal tip deprojection in open rhinoplasty. Aesthetic Plast Surg 2015;39: 53–62.

21. Patrocínio LG, Patrocínio TG, Barreto DM, et al. Evaluation of lateral crural steal in nasal tip surgery. JAMA Facial Plast Surg 2014;16(6):400–4.

22. Bared A, Rashan A, Caughlin BP, et al. Lower lateral cartilage repositioning: objective analysis using 3-dimensional imaging. JAMA Facial Plast Surg 2014;16(4):261–7.

23. Devcic Z, Rayikanti BA, Hevia JP, et al. Nasal tip projection and facial attractiveness. Laryngoscope 2011;121(7):1388–94.

24. Killian G. The submucous window resection of the nasal septum. Ann Otol Rhinol Laryngol 1905;14: 363–93.

25. Mau T, Mau ST, Kim DW. Cadaveric and engineering analysis of the septal L-strut. Laryngoscope 2007; 117(11):1902–6.

26. Stewart MG, Smith TL, Weaver EM, et al. Outcomes after nasal septoplasty: results from the nasal obstruction septoplasty effectiveness (NOSE) study. Otolaryngol Head Neck Surg 2004;130(3):283–90.

27. Metzenbaum M. Replacement of the lower end of the dislocated septal cartilage versus submucous resection of the dislocated end of the septal cartilage. Arch Otolaryngol 1929;9:282–96.

28. Haack J, Papel ID. Caudal septal deviation. Otolaryngol Clin North Am 2009;42(3):427–36.

29. Ellis M. Suture technique for caudal septal deviations. Laryngoscope 1980;90:1510–2.

30. Digman RO. Correction of nasal deformities due to defects of the septum. Plast Reconstr Surg 1956; 18:291–304.

31. Chung YS, Seol JH, Choi JM, et al. How to resolve the caudal septal deviation? Clinical outcomes after septoplasty with bony batten grafting. Laryngoscope 2014;124(8):1771–6.

32. Gubisch W. Twenty-five years experience with extracorporeal septoplasty. Facial Plast Surg 2006;22(4): 230–9.

33. Most SP. Anterior septal reconstruction: outcomes after a modified extracorporeal septoplasty technique. Arch Facial Plast Surg 2006;8(3):202–7.

34. Lee SB, Jang YJ. Treatment outcomes of extracorporeal septoplasty compared with in situ septal correction in rhinoplasty. JAMA Facial Plast Surg 2014;16(5):328–34.

35. Surowitz J, Lee MK, Most SP. Anterior septal reconstruction for treatment of severe caudal septal deviation: clinical severity and outcomes. Otolaryngol Head Neck Surg 2015. [Epub ahead of print].

36. Mabry RL. Surgery of the inferior turbinates: how much and when? Otolaryngol Head Neck Surg 1984;92:571–6.

37. Ercan C, Imre A, Pinar E, et al. Comparison of submucosal resection and radiofrequency turbinate volume reduction for inferior turbinate hypertrophy: evaluation by magnetic resonance imaging. Indian J Otolaryngol Head Neck Surg 2014;66(3):281–6.

38. Spielberg W. The treatment of nasal obstruction by submucous resection of the inferior turbinate bone. Report of cases. Laryngoscope 1924;34:197–203.

39. Hegazy HM, ElBadawey MR, Behery A. Inferior turbinate reduction; coblation versus microdebrider - a prospective, randomised study. Rhinology 2014; 52(4):306–14.

40. Aksoy F, Yıldırım YS, Veyseller B, et al. Midterm outcomes of outfracture of the inferior turbinate. Otolaryngol Head Neck Surg 2010;143(4):579–84.

41. Cavaliere M, Mottola G, Iemma M. Monopolar and bipolar radiofrequency thermal ablation of inferior turbinates: 20-month follow-up. Otolaryngol Head Neck Surg 2007;137(2):256–63.

42. Harrill WC, Pillsbury HC 3rd, McGuirt WF, et al. Radiofrequency turbinate reduction: a NOSE evaluation. Laryngoscope 2007;117(11):1912–9.

43. Havel M, Sroka R, Leunig A, et al. A double-blind, randomized, intra-individual controlled feasibility trial comparing the use of 1,470 and 940 nm diode laser for the treatment of hyperplastic inferior nasal turbinates. Lasers Surg Med 2011;43:881.

44. Gindros G, Kantas I, Balatsouras DG, et al. Comparison of ultrasound turbinate reduction, radiofrequency tissue ablation and submucosal cauterization in inferior turbinate hypertrophy. Eur Arch Otorhinolaryngol 2010;267:1723–33.

45. Batra PS, Seiden AM, Smith TL. Surgical management of adult inferior turbinate hypertrophy: a systematic review of the evidence. Laryngoscope 2009;119(9):1819–27.

46. Spielmann PM, White PS, Hussain SS. Surgical techniques for the treatment of nasal valve collapse: a systematic review. Laryngoscope 2009;119(7): 1281–90.

47. Rhee JS, Arganbright JM, McMullin BT, et al. Evidence supporting functional rhinoplasty or nasal valve repair: a 25-year systematic review. Otolaryngol Head Neck Surg 2008;139(1):10–20.

48. Andre RF, Vuyk HD. Reconstruction of dorsal and/or caudal nasal septum deformities with septal battens or by septal replacement: an overview and comparison of techniques. Laryngoscope 2006; 116:1668–73.

49. Ricci E, Palonta F, Preti G, et al. Role of nasal valve in the surgically corrected nasal respiratory obstruction: evaluation through rhinomanometry. Am J Rhinol 2001;15:307–10.

50. Toriumi DM, Josen J, Weinberger M, et al. Use of alar batten grafts for correction of nasal valve collapse. Arch Otolaryngol Head Neck Surg 1997;123(8):802–8.

51. Chand MS, Toriumi DM. Treatment of the external nasal valve. Facial Plast Surg Clin North Am 1999; 7(3):347–55.

52. Roofe SB, Most SP. Placement of a lateral nasal suspension suture via an external rhinoplasty approach. Arch Facial Plast Surg 2007;9(3): 214–6.

53. Paniello RC. Nasal valve suspension: an effective treatment for nasal valve collapse. Arch Otolaryngol Head Neck Surg 1996;122(12):1342–6.

54. Lieberman DM, Most SP. Lateral nasal wall suspension using a bone-anchored suture technique. Arch Facial Plast Surg 2010;12(2):113.

An Evidence-Based Approach to Facial Reanimation

Nate Jowett, MD*, Tessa A. Hadlock, MD

KEYWORDS

- Facial palsy • Facial paralysis • Facial reanimation • Evidence-based medicine • Synkinesis

KEY POINTS

- Management of facial palsy (FP) is dictated by the pattern and time course of dysfunction.
- Therapeutic options include pharmaceutical agents, corneal protective measures, physical therapy (PT), chemodenervation agents, fillers, and a myriad of surgical procedures.
- Good evidence from well-designed studies supports the use of glucocorticoids and antivirals in the setting of idiopathic and acute viral FP and botulinum toxin (BTX) and PT in the setting of synkinesis.
- A plethora of surgical techniques and their respective outcomes have been described in the literature, but few use controls, blinded assessment, and validated scales to reduce bias.
- Outcomes research in facial paralysis should comprise standardized subjective quality-of-life (QOL) and objective functional measures.

INTRODUCTION/OVERVIEW

Whether congenital or acquired, FP is a devastating condition with functional and aesthetic sequelae resulting in profound psychosocial and QOL impairment.[1,2] When acquired, the inciting insult typically results in acute flaccid facial palsy (FFP). Long-term functional outcomes range from full return of normal function to persistent and complete FFP. In between these extremes exist zonal permutations of hypoactivity and hyperactivity and synkinesis; such patterns of dysfunction may collectively be referred to as nonflaccid facial palsy (NFFP).[3] To reduce ambiguity,[4] a summary of pertinent definitions is provided in **Table 1**.

When severe, FFP results in loss of static and dynamic facial symmetry, brow ptosis that obscures vision, paralytic lagophthalmos resulting in exposure keratitis, collapse of the external nasal valve (ENV) impairing nasal breathing, oral incompetence, and articulation impairment. Management is focused on eye protection, restoration of symmetry at rest, and dynamic reanimation. Synkinesis-related symptoms predominate in NFFP, with periocular synkinesis resulting in a narrowed palpebral fissure width that impairs peripheral vision, midfacial synkinesis restricting meaningful smile, and platysmal synkinesis resulting in neck discomfort and facial fatigue. Efforts are concentrated on improving dynamic symmetry.

THERAPEUTIC OPTIONS AND SURGICAL TECHNIQUES

Therapeutic options for FP are dictated by the pattern and time course of dysfunction and may include pharmaceutical agents, corneal protective measures, PT, chemodenervation agents, fillers, and a myriad of surgical procedures. Patients may be classified into 1 of 5 domains: acute FFP, FFP with potential for spontaneous recovery (PSR), persistent FFP with viable or nonviable facial musculature, and NFFP. **Fig. 1** summarizes

Division of Facial Plastic and Reconstructive Surgery, Department of Otolaryngology, Facial Nerve Center, Massachusetts Eye and Ear Infirmary, Harvard Medical School, 243 Charles Street, Boston, MA 02114, USA
* Corresponding author.
E-mail address: nathan_jowett@meei.harvard.edu

Facial Plast Surg Clin N Am 23 (2015) 313–334
http://dx.doi.org/10.1016/j.fsc.2015.04.005
1064-7406/15/$ – see front matter © 2015 Elsevier Inc. All rights reserved.

Table 1
Relevant definitions

Term	Definition
Facial palsy	Term encompassing entire spectrum of facial movement disorders including facial paralysis, flaccid facial palsy, and nonflaccid facial palsy
Facial paralysis	Complete absence of facial movement and tone
Flaccid facial palsy	Absence or weakness of facial movement and tone, without synkinesis or hyperactivity
Nonflaccid facial palsy	A postparetic state whereby aberrant nerve regeneration has occurred, consisting of varying degrees of zonal synkinesis and hypoactivity and hyperactivity
Facial synkinesis	Involuntary and abnormal facial muscle activation accompanying volitional or spontaneous expression

the therapeutic options by zone and side for FFP and NFFP.

The acute setting comprises the first few weeks following onset of FFP whereby medical therapy (immunosuppressants, antivirals, and/or antibiotics), surgical decompression, or neuroplasty may be indicated. Eye lubrication and taping of the eye closed at night is indicated if paralytic lagophthalmos is present to prevent exposure keratopathy, in addition to PT for patient education and upper eyelid stretching to aid passive closure. Correction of paralytic lagophthalmos may be achieved by tarsorrhaphy or by placement of an eyelid spring or weight. Indications include poor prognosis for rapid recovery, inadequate Bell phenomenon, and absent recovery at 3 months.[5] Where nerve continuity is believed to be intact in the setting of FFP, for example, following resection of a vestibular schwannoma (VS) where FN stimulation was achieved before closure, a PSR exists with a plateau expected by 9 to 12 months.[6] Other than corneal protective measures, observation during this period is warranted.

When paralysis persists after nerve insult, native facial musculature is believed to remain receptive to reinnervation for up to 2 years after denervation. During this period, dynamic reanimation procedures using native facial musculature are possible, such as direct repair or interposition grafting of FN stumps (in the setting of an accessible FN discontinuity) or nerve transfer to the distal FN stump or specific branches (where the proximal FN is inaccessible or nonviable). Coaptation of a portion of the ipsilateral hypoglossal nerve to the entire distal FN stump restores resting tone to the face, whereas targeted nerve transfers aim to restore specific volitional facial movements such as smile or blink by coaptation of the donor nerve to the specific distal FN branch controlling the muscle of interest. Common donor nerves for targeted

transfer include branches of the contralateral FN (cross-face nerve grafting [CFNG]) or ipsilateral branches of the trigeminal nerve.

When reinnervation of the facial musculature is not possible, therapeutic options in long-standing FFP, in addition to PT and corneal protective measures, include static zonal suspensions, lower eyelid tightening, and dynamic smile reanimation. Targeted suspensions of the brow, lower eyelid, midface, nasal valve, nasolabial fold (NLF), and oral commissure may be achieved using sutures, fascia lata, and bioabsorbable or permanent implants. Tightening of the lower lid may be achieved by the lateral tarsal strip (LTS) procedure[7] with or without medical canthal tendon plication. Dynamic smile reanimation may be achieved through antidromic[8] or orthodromic[9] temporalis muscle transfer or free muscle transfer[10,11] with motor innervation provided through cranial nerve transfer. Such procedures may be paired with weakening of the normal-side brow or lip depressors or the use of fillers to efface the healthy NLF. Options for dynamic reanimation of the lower lip include anterior digastric muscle transfer,[12] CFNG or split hypoglossal neurotization of the depressor muscles or transferred digastric muscle,[13] and inlay of a T-shaped fascia graft.[14]

NFFP is by definition a chronic condition with intact yet aberrantly reinnervated facial musculature. Lagophthalmos in NFFP is exceedingly rare. PT is first-line treatment; a comprehensive program includes patient education, soft-tissue mobilization, mirror and electromyography (EMG) biofeedback, and neuromuscular retraining.[15] Blunting of hyperactivity through filler injection and weakening of hyperactive muscles through targeted chemodenervation, neurectomy, or resection in advanced disease is indicated in conjunction with PT. In cases with severe restriction of oral commissure excursion, regional

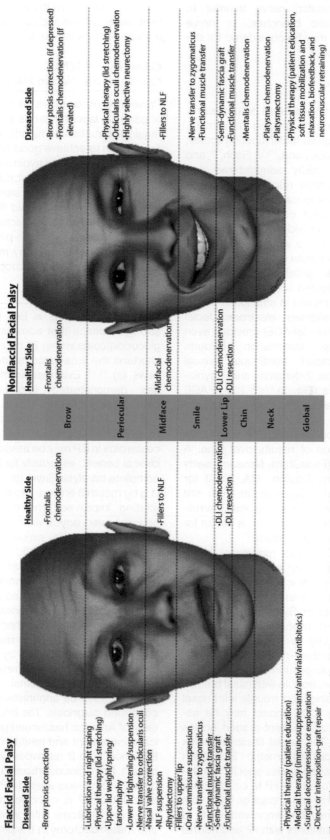

Flaccid Facial Palsy

Diseased Side
- Brow ptosis correction

- Lubrication and night taping
- Physical therapy (lid stretching)
- Upper lid weight/spring/ tarsorrhaphy
- Lower lid tightening/suspension
- Nerve transfer to orbicularis oculi
- Nasal valve correction
- NLF suspension
- Rhytidectomy
- Fillers to upper lip
- Oral commissure suspension
- Nerve transfer to zygomaticus
- Functional muscle transfer
- Semi-dynamic fascia graft
- Functional muscle transfer

- Physical therapy (patient education)
- Medical therapy (immunosuppressants/antivirals/antibiotics)
- Surgical decompression or exploration
- Direct or interposition-graft repair

Healthy Side
- Frontalis chemodenervation

- Fillers to NLF

- DLI chemodenervation
- DLI resection

Nonflaccid Facial Palsy

Healthy Side
- Frontalis chemodenervation

- Midfacial chemodenervation

- DLI chemodenervation
- DLI resection

Diseased Side
- Brow ptosis correction (if depressed)
- Frontalis chemodenervation (if elevated)

- Physical therapy (lid stretching)
- Orbicularis oculi chemodenervation
- Highly selective neurectomy

- Fillers to NLF

- Nerve transfer to zygomaticus
- Functional muscle transfer

- Semi-dynamic fascia graft
- Functional muscle transfer

- Mentalis chemodenervation

- Platysma chemodenervation
- Platysmectomy

- Physical therapy (patient education, soft tissue mobilization and relaxation, biofeedback, and neuromuscular retraining)

Brow

Periocular

Midface

Smile

Lower Lip

Chin

Neck

Global

Fig. 1. Therapeutic options for flaccid and nonflaccid facial palsy. DLI, depressor labii inferioris; NLF, nasolabial fold.

innervated muscle transfer, nerve transfer to diseased-side zygomatic branches, or nerve transfer to free muscle may be considered for dynamic smile reanimation.

CLINICAL OUTCOMES

Assessment and reporting of facial outcomes requires a robust means of grading movement. Although 5- or 6-point gross facial function scales, such as the House-Brackmann,[16,17] Fisch,[18] and others,[19,20] may be rapidly administered and demonstrate high interrater reliability, they lack the resolution necessary to capture spontaneous or treatment-related zonal changes over time. The Yanagihara scale[21] provides Likert-scale resolution of zonal appearance with movement but not at rest and lacks separate grading of synkinesis. The Sunnybrook facial grading system (FGS)[22,23] provides weighted scores of zonal symmetry at rest and with motion in addition to synkinesis. A recently validated electronic facial paralysis assessment tool (eFACE) provides even more comprehensive information through weighted clinician-graded continuous visual analog scales of 5 static, 7 dynamic, and 4 synkinetic zonal parameters (**Fig. 2**).[24,25] The eFACE tool consists of a database-linked graphical user interface designed for rapid administration using a touch-screen device allowing for immediate graphical representation of results over time. A freeware Java applet (FaceGram, Massachusetts Eye and Ear Infirmary, Boston, MA, USA) for scaled semiautomated measurements from still images of facial parameters, such as oral commissure excursion and philtral deviation, is useful for quantitative analysis of interventions.[26]

In addition to grading facial movement, standardized assessments of FP-related symptoms and QOL are necessary to track the burden of disease and response to interventions. The patient-graded Nasal Obstruction Symptom Evaluation (NOSE)[27] instrument is useful in patients with ENV collapse secondary to FFP.[28] The NOSE scale consists of patient-reported symptom scores for nasal congestion or stuffiness, blockage or obstruction, trouble with nasal breathing, trouble with sleeping, and trouble with nasal breathing on exertion. QOL impact may be assessed using generalized patient-graded scales such as the SF-36.[29] The Facial Disability Index (FDI)[30] and the Facial Clinimetric Evaluation (FaCE)[1] are patient-graded scales specifically designed and validated for use in FP to concurrently assess symptom severity and impact on QOL, with the FaCE scale demonstrating improved ability to discriminate between patients with FP and normal controls. **Figs. 3–10** illustrate a wide range of patient presentations and clinical outcomes following therapeutic interventions.

CLINICAL EVIDENCE
Corneal Protection in Flaccid Facial Palsy

Prevention of exposure keratopathy in the setting of paralytic lagophthalmos is paramount. Patients require instruction on nighttime ointment and tape application to achieve good adherence of the tape to the upper eyelid, to avoid inadvertent eye opening and potential corneal abrasion from the tape itself (level V).[31] For the same reason, patients should be advised to avoid the direct placement of a soft patch over the affected eye. Emerging evidence indicates that a gas-permeable scleral lens worn up to 12 hours a day may be used to treat and prevent exposure keratopathy (level IV).[32,33]

Pharmaceutical Therapy

When the diagnosis is Bell palsy (BP), there is strong evidence that administration of high-dose glucocorticoids within 72 hours of symptom onset shortens the time to complete recovery in adults (level Ia).[34,35] Evidence from subgroup analysis has demonstrated improved outcomes for prednisone-equivalent doses totaling 450 mg or higher.[36] Antiviral monotherapy is contraindicated (level Ib).[37,38] Combined use of antivirals and corticosteroids in BP may be associated with additional clinical benefit, especially for those with severe to complete paralysis (level Ib),[36,39] with valacyclovir (1 g by mouth 3 times a day for 7–10 days) demonstrating improved time to resolution of acute neuritis over acyclovir.[40] Combination therapy should be used in varicella-zoster virus (VZV)-associated FP (level IV).[41,42] When FP follows trauma or surgery, it is prudent to use glucocorticoids; however, only noncontrolled case series (level IV) have been reported on their use.[43,44]

Common infectious causes of FP include Lyme disease and acute otitis media (AOM). FP occurs in 8% of cases of Lyme disease meeting diagnostic criteria established by the Centers for Disease Control and Prevention.[45] Targeted antibiotic therapy against Borrelia burgdorferi should always be administered in the setting of a confirmed diagnosis. The Infectious Diseases Society of America has issued guidelines for the clinical assessment and treatment of Lyme disease.[46] Evidence from 2 retrospective studies reveals no benefit from glucocorticoid use in the setting of Lyme disease–associated FP (level IV).[47,48] AOM-associated FP is managed with targeted antibiotics, myringotomy with or without tube insertion, and mastoidectomy in the presence of coalescent

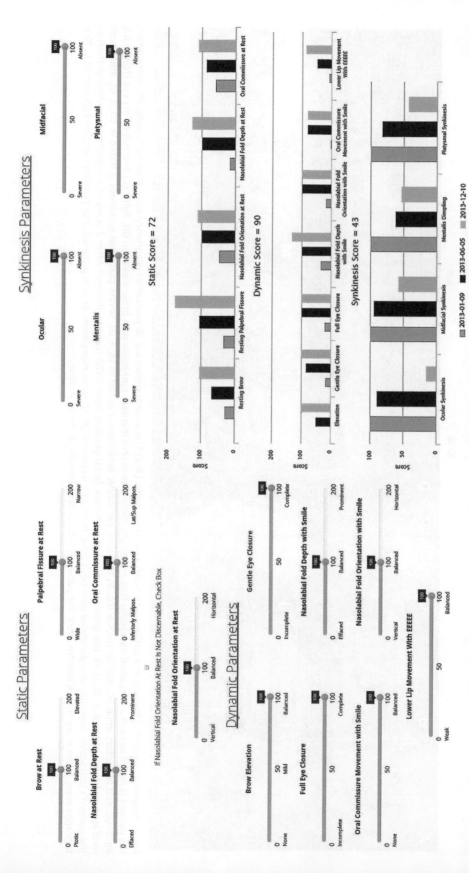

Fig. 2. The eFACE graphical user interface (GUI). Static (*top left*), dynamic (*bottom left*), and synkinesis (*top right*) parameters are assessed. Once entered, the GUI allows for immediate visual comparison with previous scores (*bar chart, bottom right*).

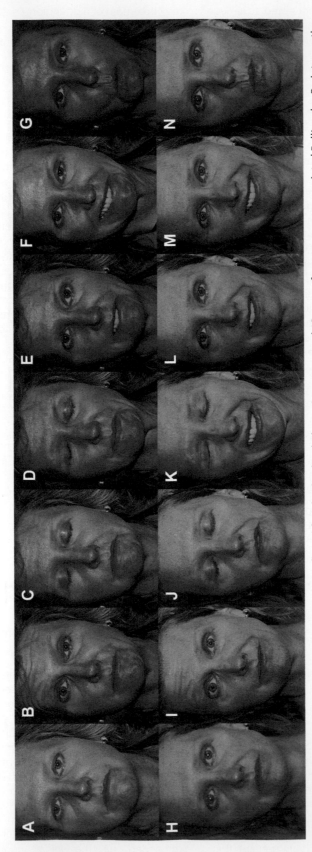

Fig. 3. Response to physical therapy in a patient with nonflaccid facial palsy. (*Top*) The patient presented 18 years after pregnancy-associated Bell's palsy. Preintervention, the patient is noted to have a deepened nasolabial fold at rest (*A*), moderate-severe mentalis synkinesis with brow elevation (*B*), light- (*C*) and full-effort eye closure (*D*), light- (*E*) and full-effort smile (*F*), and lip pucker (*G*). In addition, periocular synkinesis is noted in (*B*, *F*, *G*), severe platysmal synkinesis is noted in (*D*, *F*, *G*), and severe midfacial synkinesis is noted in (*B*, *D*, *F*). Her preintervention Sunnybrook facial grading score (FGS) was 54. (*Bottom*) After 2 years of comprehensive physical therapy, the patient's periocular, mentalis, and platysmal synkinesis have markedly improved (*H–N*, same expressions as in top panel). Her postintervention FGS was 71.5. Photographs were taken more than 6 months after the patient's most recent botulinum toxin A dose.

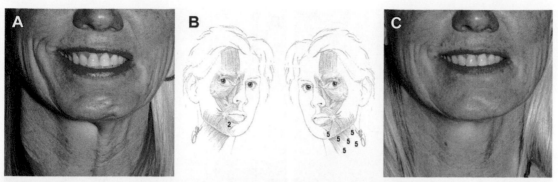

Fig. 4. Botulinum toxin (BTX) for platysmal synkinesis. The patient developed nonflaccid facial palsy 20 years previously after resection of a vestibular schwannoma. (*A*) Marked platysmal banding and mentalis dimpling with restriction of oral commissure excursion on the patients left side is demonstrated before treatment. (*B*) The patient was injected with 2 units of BTX-A to the contralateral depressor labii inferioris, 5 units to the ipsilateral side of the mentalis, and 25 units to the ipsilateral platysma. (*C*) Four weeks after injection, platysmal banding and mentalis dimpling have significantly resolved, and smile is more symmetric.

mastoiditis (level IV).[49,50] When contraindications such as diabetes mellitus are not present, glucocorticoid use in AOM-associated FP is recommended based on case series (level IV)[49,50]; however, no controlled studies could be found in the literature.

Surgical Exploration and Decompression in Acute Flaccid Facial Palsy

Evidence has shown that spontaneous return of satisfactory (House-Brackmann grade [HBG] I or II) facial function following BP is reduced by 50% when electroneuronography (ENoG) reveals a

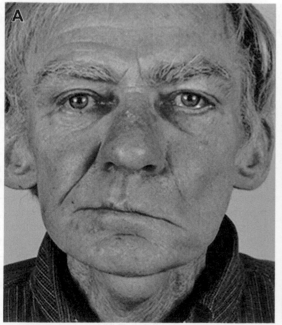
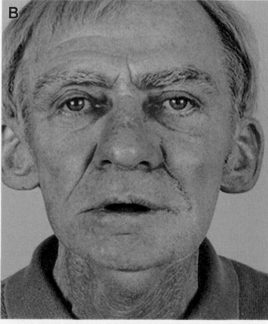

Fig. 5. Static 3-ribbon fascia lata suspension. (*A*) The patient developed flaccid facial paralysis subsequent to an invasive parotid gland carcinoma. Midfacial ptosis with effacement of the nasal labial fold and inferior malposition of the oral commissure at rest are noted on the patient's left side. (*B*) Following static suspension using 3 strips of fascia lata to suspend the ipsilateral nasal alar base, the nasolabial fold, and the oral commissure, facial symmetry is improved at rest.

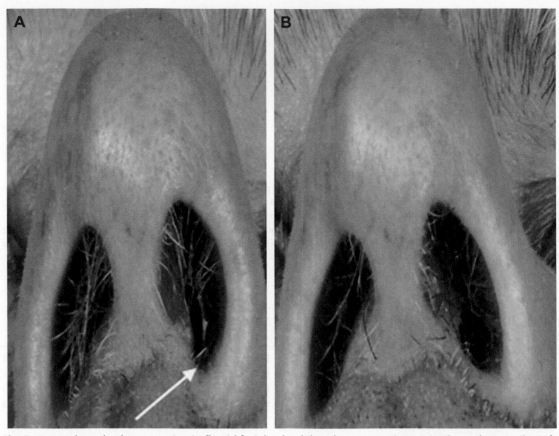

Fig. 6. External nasal valve correction in flaccid facial palsy. (*A*) In the same patient as in **Fig. 4**, the nostril is inferiorly and medially displaced resulting in blunting of the nasal vestibule in the region of the nasal sill (*arrow*). (*B*) Following static suspension of the alar base using fascia lata secured to the temporalis fascia, the nostril is pulled superiorly and laterally with subsequent correction of the nasal vestibule collapse.

greater than 95% difference between sides within 2 weeks of symptom onset.[18] In that prospective controlled (level IIb) study by Fisch,[18] a 30% or greater improvement in satisfactory outcomes in this cohort of patients was achieved when decompression of the site of pathologic constriction, the meatal foramen in 94% of cases, together with neighboring segments via a middle cranial fossa approach was completed within 24 hours of the point where serial ENoG demonstrated 90% to 94% degeneration. A second prospective controlled (level IIb) trial confirmed that surgical decompression that included the meatal foramen resulted in a clinically and statistically significant improvement in long-term outcomes for patients with a diagnosis of BP presenting with severe or complete flaccid paralysis (ie, HBG V or VI), an ENoG response demonstrating greater than 90% degeneration compared with the contralateral healthy side, and absence of voluntary motor unity potentials on EMG.[51] In that study by Gantz and colleagues,[51] 91% of patients meeting the

inclusion criteria who underwent decompression within 2 weeks of symptom onset in addition to medical therapy progressed to a final HBG of I or II, compared with 42% of patients who received medical therapy alone (*P* = .0002) (level IIb). Both studies were biased by patient self-selection for surgery; this limitation, together with the technical difficulty and associated risks of decompression surgery, such as hearing loss, cerebrospinal leak, and iatrogenic facial nerve injury, prevents consensus on its utilization.[35] Although May and colleagues[52,53] have advocated that decompression is of no benefit in BP, their conclusions were based on a transmastoid approach in which the meatal foramen was not decompressed.[51]

Others have extended the indications for decompression in BP to VZV-associated[44] and delayed traumatic FFP[43,44,54,55] (level IV), with weak evidence demonstrating benefit even when surgery is delayed by more than 3 weeks (level IV).[44,54,55] Exploration is indicated when

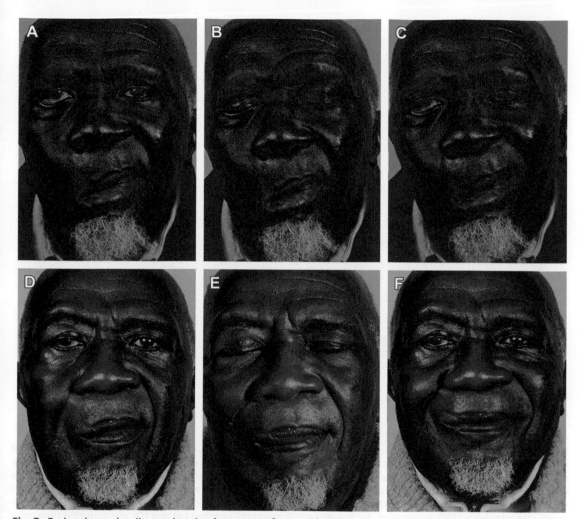

Fig. 7. Periocular and smile reanimation by means of an antidromic temporalis muscle transfer. (*Top*) The patient presented with complete FFP 2 years after an attempt at interposition graft repair of ballistic trauma to the patient's right facial nerve. Brow ptosis, lateral canthal tendon laxity with scleral show and ectropion, and significant midfacial and oral commissure ptosis are seen at rest (*A*). Eye closure is incomplete with light effort (*B*), and no movement is seen with smile on the affected side (*C*). (*Bottom*) The patient underwent ipsilateral brow ptosis correction, platinum upper eyelid weight insertion, lateral tarsal strip procedure, and an antidromic temporalis muscle transfer. Facial symmetry is markedly improved at rest (*D*), eye closure is complete with light effort (*E*), and dynamic smile is restored with bite (*F*).

immediate and unexpected FP arises following surgery in the region of the nerve (level V)[56] and has been advocated in cases in which temporal bone fracture results in immediate facial paralysis, under the assumption that immediate onset indicates nerve transection or impalement by bone fragments. Only noncontrolled case series (level IV)[43,54] appear in the literature, demonstrating clinical benefit with exploration in the setting of immediate-onset traumatic FP. When combined with the fact that coexisting trauma and neurologic impairment often make it difficult to ascertain whether paralysis is immediate or delayed, the lack of clear evidence indicating benefit leaves

the role of surgical exploration and decompression in the setting of temporal trauma unclear.[57]

Observation and Timing of Interventions

Evidence from large retrospective case series has shown that even without treatment, 70% of patients with BP fully recover (ie, HBG 1), 15% recover with only minor deficits (ie, HBG II), and 15% progress to NFFP (ie, HBG III–IV).[53,58] Persistence of severe or complete FFP (ie, HBG V or VI) in BP does not occur. Evidence from a large retrospective case series has demonstrated that following VS resection with anatomically intact

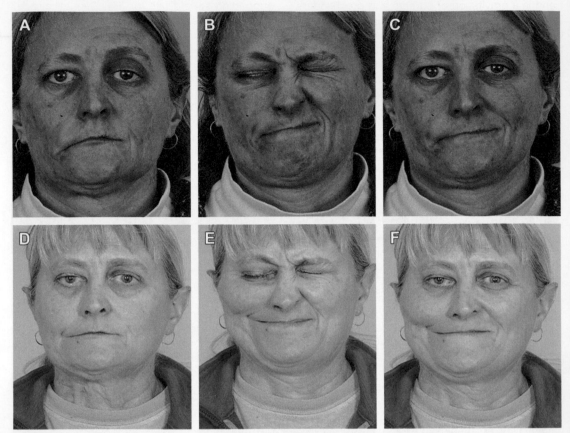

Fig. 8. Free-gracilis transfer with cross-face nerve graft (CFNG) innervation. (*Top*) The patient presented at age 50 years with symptoms present since birth and opted for spontaneous smile reanimation despite the risks of a poor result. Before any intervention, brow, lower lid, and midfacial ptosis are noted (*A*), with incomplete eye closure with full effort (*B*) and lack of meaningful commissure excursion with smile on the patient's right side (*C*). (*Bottom*) Following brow ptosis correction, lateral tarsal strip procedure, platinum eyelid weight insertion, and 2-stage free gracilis transfer with CFNG innervation, facial symmetry is markedly improved at rest (*D*), eye closure is now complete with full effort (*E*), and spontaneous smile with excellent and symmetric excursion is achieved (*F*).

FNs, 94% being via the retrosigmoid approach, all patients with an initial postoperative HBG of III or IV recover without significant deficit (ie, to an HBG of I or II) within 6 to 12 months (level IV).[6] In that same study by Rivas and colleagues,[6] patients having a persistent postoperative HBG of VI at 7 months were noted to have at least an 80% probability of a poor outcome (ie, HBG IV,V, or VI), with this probability approaching 100% by 9 months (level IV), supporting early nerve transfer interventions while facial musculature is still receptive to reinnervation.

Neurorrhaphy

Nerve transections necessitate decision making with regards to timing of repair, need for interposition grafting, and coaptation technique. Following denervation, it has been demonstrated in animal models that neuromuscular junctions become progressively less receptive to regenerating motor axons.[59–61] Evidence from case series suggests that the time to reinnervation is likely the most important factor and that delays longer than 12 to 24 months result in significantly worse mimetic outcomes (level IV).[62–64] Increasing age has also been shown to result in decreasing capacity for neuron survival, neural regeneration, and/or muscle receptivity to reinnervation following injury in animal models.[65–68] It follows that reconnection of viable motor axons to facial musculature should proceed without delay in the setting of known neural discontinuity. When presentation is delayed or when no recovery of function occurs following injury not resulting in transection, no definitive criteria exist for predicting the degree to which the facial musculature remains receptive to reinnervation.[61] Postoperative radiation therapy has

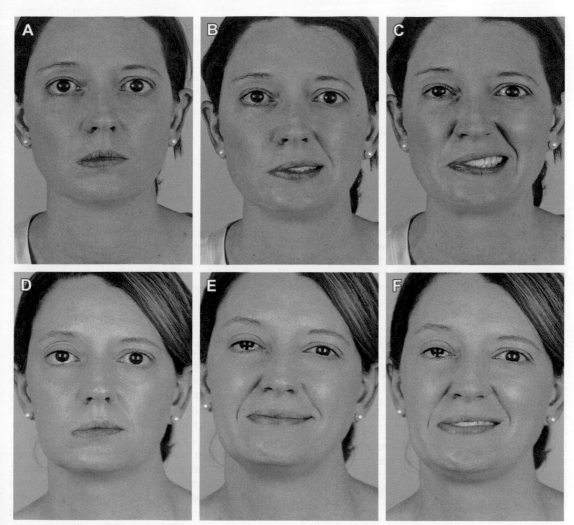

Fig. 9. Trigeminal-to-facial nerve (V-VII) transfer. (*Top*) The patient presented 2 years after interposition grafting of the proximal right facial nerve following tumor extirpation. At rest, mild hyperelevation of the brow and effacement of the nasolabial fold is noted (*A*). Light- (*B*) and full-effort smile (*C*) demonstrate limited commissure excursion on the affected side. (*Bottom*) Following V-VII transfer and contralateral depressor labii inferioris chemodenervation, facial appearance is unchanged at rest (*D*), and smile symmetry with light- (*E*) and full-effort smile (*F*) is markedly improved.

been shown to have negligible impact on neural regeneration and ultimate mimetic outcomes in animal models[69] and in clinical case series[70–72] (level IV); as such, it should play no role in decision making with regards to neurorrhaphy.

Many surgeons use a threshold gap of 5 mm to prompt the use of an interposition graft. Evidence from animal studies demonstrates a clear inverse relationship between tension across the repair site and outcomes[73–78]; better outcomes are achieved using a cable graft of suitable diameter when direct end-to-end repair would result in a tension exceeding 0.3 to 0.4 N across defects 6 mm or greater.[73,75] Although many surgeons

inlay grafts in reverse polarity, based on the presumption that this results in fewer regenerating axons being lost along exiting branches, evidence for this practice is lacking; most animal studies have shown no dependency of electrophysiologic, histologic, or functional outcome measures on graft polarity.[79–81] One animal study demonstrated decreased graft cross-sectional area with orthodromic compared with antidromic positioning[82]; however, this study was severely limited by lack of functional outcomes measures and axonal counts. Clinical case series have demonstrated worse facial nerve functional outcomes with interposition grafting in older patients than

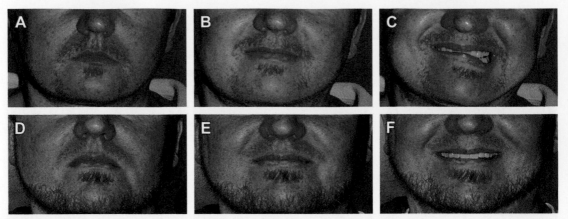

Fig. 10. Trigeminal-to-facial nerve (V-VII) transfer. (*Top*) The patient presented with a remote history of isolated iatrogenic marginal-mandibular nerve transection. Facial symmetry is noted at rest (*A*) and with light-effort smile (*B*). Marked asymmetry is noted with full-effort smile due to contralateral (healthy side) depressor labii inferioris (DLI) activation in this patient with a full-denture smile (*C*). (*Bottom*) After a trial of DLI chemodenervation, the patient opted for DLI resection. Symmetry is now demonstrated at rest (*D*) and with light- (*E*) and full-effort smile (*F*).

in younger patients (<30–60 years of age) (level IV).[71,72]

Coaptation technique is an important consideration. Evidence from animal models has demonstrated no statistical difference in functional or electrophysiologic outcomes between interfascicular and epineurial neurorrhaphy following transection.[83–88] Histologic studies have demonstrated increased neuroma lengths at neurorrhaphy sites resulting from interfascicular compared with epineurial repair without statistical difference in myelinated fiber counts between groups in the distal segment 12 months following repair.[89] Use of fibrin adhesive in comparison with microsutures for nerve transection repair and cable graft coaptation has demonstrated equivalent functional and long-term histologic outcomes in the vast majority of randomized controlled studies in animal models while offering the advantage of reduced operating time[90–103]; however, a minority of studies have demonstrated statistically inferior electrophysiologic outcomes,[104,105] with one demonstrating decreased axon counts[106] in the case in which fibrin glue was used as opposed to nylon microsutures. High-quality human studies comparing coaptation using fibrin glue with conventional epineurial suture repair are lacking; retrospective reviews have demonstrated equivalent functional outcomes for fibrin glue repair of brachial plexus and digital nerves (level IV)[107] and the facial nerve.[108,109] Cyanoacrylate should not be used for nerve coaptation, as it causes a profound foreign-body inflammatory reaction and subsequent fibrosis (level V).[110]

Physiotherapy

Despite the conclusions of a 2011 meta-analysis,[111] good evidence supports the use of PT in FP. In a randomized controlled trial (RCT) by Beurskens and colleagues,[112,113] patients with long-standing NFFP following BP, AN resection, VZV infection, and trauma receiving 3 months of comprehensive facial PT as opposed to being waitlisted demonstrated statistical improvements in patient-reported facial stiffness and FDI scores and quantitative assessment of lip length; however, no statistical benefit was seen in blinded expert-assessed FGS scores 12 months after therapy (level Ib). In the 2014 RCT by Pourmomeny and colleagues,[114] patients with acute FFP (onset within 3 weeks) resulting from BP, trauma, or tumor extraction who received PT that included EMG biofeedback demonstrated significantly improved FGS scores at 1 year compared with those receiving PT without EBF (77 ± 16 vs 56 ± 27, $P<.05$); however, those assessing FGS were not blinded (level Ib). In that same study, further assessment by 1 blinded reviewer of synkinesis based on a custom scale demonstrated that 31% of patients who received PT that included EBF demonstrated moderate to severe synkinesis at 1 year compared with 77% of patients who received PT that did not include EBF (relative risk, 0.41, 95% confidence interval, 0.19–0.89) (level Ib).[114] An RCT by Nicastri and colleagues[115] demonstrated that 74% of patients with BP presenting with severe to complete FFP (ie, HBG V/VI) who received combination pharmacologic therapy (CPT) with prednisone and valacyclovir plus comprehensive PT within 10 days of symptom onset progressed to an HBG of I or II as assessed by 1 blinded expert within 6 months, compared with only 48% of those receiving CPT alone (adjusted P = .038) (level Ib). In summary, recent evidence supports the use of PT in acute FFP and long-standing NFFP.

INJECTABLES

Chemodenervation has become a mainstay of treatment in NFFP and an adjunctive treatment in FFP. A placebo-controlled, double-blinded, and presumably randomized trial comparing BTX to saline injection into synkinetic zones of patients with NFFP following BP, AN resection, VZV infection, mastoiditis, and meningioma resection demonstrated statistically significant improvements in synkinesis scores using a custom ordinal grading scale from 0 (none) to 6 (very severe) as assessed by 1 blinded expert for those receiving BT versus saline placebo (0.467 ± 1.06 vs 4.42 ± 1.42, $P<.001$) (level Ib).[116] Blinded patient-reported measures of overall QOL, social functioning, personal appearance, visual function, and synkinesis severity demonstrated significant postinjection improvements for those in the BT treatment arm ($P<.05$, all measures) but not for saline placebo group ($P>.05$, all measures). Evidence from case series has demonstrated that in patients with flaccid paralysis, BT injection to the contralateral lip depressors improves lower-lip symmetry,[117] that injection into the contralateral NLF region improves oral competence,[118] and that injection into the contralateral forehead improves brow symmetry (level IV).[119] In addition, injectable fillers, such as hyaluronic acid, hydroxyapatite, and fat grafts, may be beneficial in the midface and lips (level V).[5]

Surgery

Brow

Correction of the ptotic brow may be achieved through open or minimally invasive means. Takushima and colleagues[120] found that, based on quantitative preoperative and 1-year postoperative anthropometric measurements of brow height, use of the endoscopic brow life in unilateral FFP is best suited for young patients with minor ptosis and is ineffective in elderly patients with severe ptosis (level IV). Ueda and colleagues[121] found that after a minimum of 3 years, symmetric positioning of the eyebrow was maintained in 26 of 40 (65%) and visual field improvement in 34 of 40 (85%) patients undergoing a unilateral direct brow lift for FFP (level IV). A recently described minimally invasive approach, which uses heavy sutures tunneled through stab incisions at the eyebrow secured to a titanium miniplate through a small pretrichial incision, found an averaged sustained suspension of 5.7 mm at follow-up (12–448 days) (level IV).[122]

Periocular complex

Surgical intervention is indicated in prolonged lagophthalmos. Tarsorrhaphy is indicated for prevention and treatment of exposure keratopathy, with evidence from case series demonstrating a 90% rate of complete resolution of established corneal ulceration (level IV).[123,124] The unfavorable aesthetics and light path obstruction caused by tarsorrhaphy have resulted in a preference for upper eyelid springs and weights for keratopathy prevention (level IV).[125] In comparison to weights, springs offer more closing force but are more difficult to insert, require frequent adjustments, and can migrate, weaken, or fracture with time (level IV).[126] Use of platinum weights over gold has demonstrated lower complication rates such as extrusion, astigmatism, and bulging (level IIIb),[127,128] likely the result of its decreased allergenicity and higher density, which permits the use of thinner profiles.

Lower-lid laxity and ectropion may be corrected through eyelid suspension or canthal tightening. Using a split palmaris longus tendon inserted through a subciliary tunnel to suspend the lower lid, Terzis and Kyere[129] achieved good or excellent outcome in terms of scleral show and lagophthalmos (when combined with an eyelid weight) in 47 of 58 (81%) patients (level IV). Tightening of the medial canthal tendon (MCT) may be achieved by plication and tightening of the lateral canthal tendon by the LTS procedure. In a study of periocular reconstruction in FFP, Golio and colleagues[130] found favorable outcomes in terms of decreased dependence on lubricating drops and resolution of foreign-body sensation in most of the 56 patients who had undergone LTS, in addition to gold weight and lateral tarsorrhaphy (level IV). Complications of LTS include granuloma formation, suture abscess, and dehiscence (5%–8%).[131] Lateralization of the lacrimal punctum may occur following LTS in the setting of coexisting MCT laxity; it may be avoided by concurrent MCT plication.[131]

In the setting of severe periocular synkinesis in NFFP, PT and BT may be inadequate. Partial orbicularis oculi denervation via a 2-step highly selective neurectomy has been described in a small case series with good results (level IV).[132]

Midface

Suspension of the NLF and ENV in FFP restores midfacial balance at rest and improves nasal breathing. Using 3 strips of fascia lata to suspend the ENV, NLF, and oral commissure, Bhama and colleagues[133] demonstrated a significant improvement in patient-reported FaCE scores and temporally blinded expert assessment of midfacial appearance (MFA) on a 10-point Likert scale between preoperative and postoperative periods (FaCE 45 ± 16 vs 58 ± 18, $P = .004$, respectively, and MFA 3.19 ± 2.40 vs 6.81 ± 1.60, $P = .0001$, respectively) (level IV). In a recent study of 40 patients undergoing fascia lata suspension of the NLF, Lindsay and colleagues[134] demonstrated significant improvements in NOSE scores between preoperative and postoperative periods (37.6 ± 27.1 vs 16.6 ± 17.4, $P<.001$) (level IV). In patients with short life expectancies, NLF suspension may be achieved under local anesthesia using multiple 2-0 polypropylene sutures through dermis and superficial musculoaponeurotic system (SMAS) passed subcutaneously to the temporal region using a Keith needle (level IV).[135] Although expanded polytetrafluoroethylene eliminates donor site morbidity, its use is not advised in static facial suspension because of loss of correction over time due to stretch and propensity for infection (level IV).[136]

Smile
Depending on the time course and pattern of disease, dynamic reanimation of smile may be achieved through reinnervation of native facial musculature or muscle and nerve transfer techniques. In a case series by Hadlock and colleagues[137] examining outcomes following free gracilis transfer in 17 children, mean smile excursion was 8.8 ± 5.0 mm, and FaCE QOL scores in 13 patients who completed preoperative and postoperative questionnaires improved significantly (51.3 vs 65.7, $P = .01$) (level IV). In a review of 127 free gracilis transfers by Bhama and colleagues,[138] failure rates were nonsignificantly lower and excursion lengths were significantly greater for masseteric branch of the trigeminal nerve (MBTN) than for CNFG innervated flaps (6% vs 16%, $P = .09$ and 8.7 ± 3.5 vs 6.5 ± 2.9, $P = .006$). A QOL outcomes study following free gracilis transfer for smile reanimation found significant improvement in preoperative versus postoperative FaCE scores (42.3 ± 15.9 vs 58.5 ± 17.6, $P<.001$) with higher but statistically nonsignificant scores for patients whose flaps were innervated by a CFNG as opposed to MBTN (61.7 ± 16.9 vs 55.2 ± 18.2, $P = .17$) (level IIIb).[134] A comparative study examining outcomes following smile reanimation by orthodromic temporalis tendon transfer using intervening strips of fascia lata (29 patients) against free latissimus dorsi transfer powered by

branches of the contralateral FN (11 patients) found nonsignificant differences between groups on postoperative Harii smile grade[11] (3.3 vs 3.6, $P>.05$, respectively) (level IIIb).[139] In summary, evidence supports the effectiveness of surgery in dynamic reanimation of smile with resultant improvement in patient QOL.

Lower face
Restoration of lower-lip symmetry is of aesthetic importance in FP. When favorable results are achieved by contralateral BT injection, permanent weakening of the lip depressors by surgical resection may be considered. In a study by Hussain and colleagues[140] of patients with NFFP or FFP who underwent contralateral depressor labii inferioris resection, 18 of 21 (86%) and 29 of 36 (81%) who though that their lower lip was asymmetrical either at rest or with smile, respectively, before the procedure reported significant postoperative improvements ($P<.001$) without any significant change in oral competence ($P = .147$) (level IV). When contralateral lip depressor weakening is undesirable, such as in patients with full-denture[141] smiles, Terzis and Kalantarian[13] reported significant postoperative improvements in dynamic lip depression by nonblinded expert assessment using a custom scale by CFNG or split hypoglossal transfer to native lip depressors within 12 months of denervation, CFNG to transferred ipsilateral anterior belly of digastric in long-standing FFP, and contralateral platysmal muscle transfer ($P<.05$ between preoperative and postoperative scores for all methods) (level IV). A novel semidynamic approach to lower lip reanimation in 9 patients using 2 fascia lata strips arranged in a T-shape described by Watanabe and colleagues[14] demonstrated significant improvements in physician-assessed symmetry at rest, with smiling, and during mouth opening with mean total scores on a custom scale from 0 to 7 improving from 1.43 to 5.71 ($P<.01$) (level IV).

Neck
Platysmal synkinesis is common in NFFP. In severe cases, when a favorable response to BTX chemodenervation is achieved, platysmectomy may be considered. Henstrom and colleagues[142] reported significant improvement in FaCE scores between preoperative and postoperative periods reported by 24 patients who underwent platysmectomy (46.7 vs 55.2, $P = .02$) (level IV). As platysmal fibers interdigitate with those of the lip depressors, the surgeon must counsel the patient on the potential effects of the procedure on the patient's postoperative smile.[143]

Table 2
Summary of static reanimation procedures including risks and concerns by facial zone

Region	Technique	Ideal Candidate	Specific Risks/Concerns
Brow	Endoscopic	Young, mild ptosis	Ineffective in severe ptosis and elderly patients
	Coronal	Female, short forehead	Raises the hairline, incisional alopecia, contraindicated in receding hairline/bald patients
	Pretrichial	Female, long forehead	Drops the hairline, contraindicated in receding hairline/bald patients
	Midforehead	Elderly, deep rhytids	Conspicuous scar
	Direct (supra) brow	Elderly, thick eyebrows, severe ptosis	Conspicuous scar, incisional alopecia
	Suture suspension	Short life expectancy, impaired peripheral vision or eye irritation	Brow dimpling, long-term effectiveness unclear
Upper lid	Tarsorrhaphy	Documented corneal ulceration	Obstructs vision, unfavorable cosmesis
	Eyelid spring	Patient who requires excellent eye closure	Technically challenging, requires frequent adjustments, risk of extrusion
	Eyelid weight	Patient who requires fair eye closure	Risk of extrusion, induced astigmatism, unsightly bulging (all reduced with the use of platinum over gold)
	Scleral lens	Documented corneal ulceration	Protects the cornea but does not improve cosmesis when used in isolation, difficult for patient to insert and remove
Lower lid	Lateral tarsal strip	Lateral canthal tendon laxity	Lateralization of the lacrimal punctum (avoid by performing concurrent medial canthal tendon plication), recurrent laxity
	Medial canthal tendon plication	Medial canthal tendon laxity	Recurrent laxity
Midface	Nasolabial fold suspension (fascia lata)	Older adults and elderly with FFP	Risk of suture abscess/extrusion and recurrent laxity, may be performed concurrently with dynamic smile reanimation
	Rhytidectomy	Deepened nasolabial fold (NFFP)	Hematoma, insufficient correction
Nasal base	Alar base suspension (fascia lata)	Collapsed external nasal valve	Risk of suture abscess/extrusion and recurrent laxity
Oral commissure	Commissure suspension (fascia lata)	Ptotic oral commissure	Not necessary if dynamic smile reanimation is planned
Lower lip	Contralateral DLI ± DAO resection	Good results from chemodenervation	Risk of mental nerve injury, risk of injury to FN branch to mentalis muscle, unfavorable cosmesis in some patients
	Contralateral MMFN resection	Not advised	Not advised due to weakening of mentalis resulting in mastication and oral competence impairments
Neck	Platysmectomy	Moderate to severe platysmal synkinesis	Cervical scar, hematoma, recurrence if insufficient muscle excised, effect on smile must be considered

Abbreviations: DAO, depressor anguli oris; DLI, depressor labii inferioris; MMFN, marginal-mandibular branch of the facial nerve.

Table 3
Summary of dynamic reanimation procedures including risks and concerns by facial zone

Region	Technique		Ideal Candidate	Risks/Concerns
Main FN trunk	Direct or interposition graft repair		Accessible proximal and distal stumps, denervation <18 mo	Best expected outcome is HBG III-IV
	XII-VII		Accessible distal stumps, denervation <18 mo	Best expected outcome is HBG III-IV, significant tongue morbidity, use is decreasing due to success of midfacial V-VII transfers
Periocular	CFNG		Denervation <18 mo	Low rate of success
Smile	Muscle	Native facial	Denervation <18–24 mo	Results unpredictable, less excursion (power) than temporalis or free muscle transfer
		Antidromic temporalis transfer	Nonviable facial muscle, poor candidate for free flap, thin masseter (female)	Cosmetically unfavorable (bulk over zygoma, hollowing of temporal fossa), contraindicated in edentulous patients, preoperative wasting, or trigeminal dysfunction
		Orthodromic temporalis transfer	Nonviable facial muscle, poor candidate for free flap, thick masseter (male)	Requires coronoid process osteotomy, contraindicated in edentulous patients/ preoperative wasting/ trigeminal dysfunction
		Free gracilis	Normal body mass index	Requires 2 stages if powered by CFNG, lengthy scar (10 cm), short pedicle (5–6 cm)
		Free latissimus dorsi	Patient who wants a single-stage procedure powered by contralateral cross-face	Cannot elevate flap simultaneously with recipient site preparation, bulky flap, lengthy scar
	Nerve	CFNG	Younger patients (<30 y) who prefer spontaneous smile over powerful smile	Requires 2 stages if paired with free gracilis (6-9 months between stages), risk of induced donor site weakness, fewer available motor axons, less excursion, less chance of success in patients >30 y
		MBTN	Older patients (>30 y) or those who prefer more smile excursion	Requires motor reeducation (straightforward), does not reanimate spontaneous smile, contraindicated in edentulous patients, preoperative wasting, or trigeminal dysfunction
Lower lip	Anterior belly of digastric muscle transfer		Patients with full denture smile[140]	Requires neuromuscular retraining, dynamic effect is questionable, bulkiness and long scar
	Nerve transfer (CFNG from marginal-mandibular branch or split XII)		Patients with full denture smile, denervation <18 mo	Efficacy is not well established, risk of induced donor site weakness
	Ipsilateral bidirectional fascia graft		Patients with full denture smile	Semidynamic, efficacy not well established

Abbreviations: MBTN, masseteric branch of the trigeminal nerve; V, trigeminal nerve; VII, facial nerve; XII, hypoglossal nerve.

COMPLICATIONS AND CONCERNS

Medical therapy, injections, and surgery are not without risk. Serious and even fatal complications have been associated with corticosteroid pulse therapy.[144] Reported reactions include infectious (sepsis, pneumonia), neuropsychiatric (sleep disturbances, psychosis), cardiovascular (hypertension, arrhythmias, fluid retention), metabolic (diabetes, cataracts), gastrointestinal (ulceration, bleeding), musculoskeletal (osteonecrosis of the femoral head),[145] and pulmonary (bronchospasm). Doxycycline is known to interfere with bone and tooth development and should be avoided in children younger than 8 years and in pregnant women for the treatment of Lyme disease.[46] Valacyclovir is currently listed as category B for all trimesters of pregnancy and deemed safe in lactation; however, rare anaphylactoid, hematologic, and renal side effects have been reported with its use. Although rare, spread of BTX outside the injection area may occur, resulting in dysphagia, respiratory paralysis, and death; a US Food and Drug Administration black box warning was issued in 2009. Periorbital BTX injection in NFFP may lead to induced lagophthalmos and exposure keratopathy, undesired lid ptosis, or diplopia,[116] whereas brow injection may lead to induced ptosis with subsequent visual field impairment and unfavorable cosmesis. Surgical risks and concerns are summarized in **Table 2** (static procedures) and **Table 3** (dynamic reanimation) by technique and facial zone.

SUMMARY

Therapeutic options for FP include pharmaceutical agents, corneal protective measures, PT, chemo-denervation agents, fillers, and surgical reanimation procedures. Although strong evidence from well-designed studies exists for many of the conservative options, surgical outcome studies are often biased because of lack of randomization, control arms, assessor blinding, and long-term follow-up and use of validated tools to assess therapeutic impact on facial function and QOL. Although there is little doubt of the crucial role surgery plays in improving the lives of patients with FP, higher-quality studies are necessary wherever equipoise exists to advance the field.

REFERENCES

1. Kahn JB, Gliklich RE, Boyev KP, et al. Validation of a patient-graded instrument for facial nerve paralysis: the FaCE scale. Laryngoscope 2001;111:387–98.

2. Ishii LE, Godoy A, Encarnacion CO, et al. What faces reveal: impaired affect display in facial paralysis. Laryngoscope 2011;121:1138–43.

3. Lindsay RW, Bhama P, Weinberg J, et al. The success of free gracilis muscle transfer to restore smile in patients with nonflaccid facial paralysis. Ann Plast Surg 2014;73:177–82.

4. Linder TE, Abdelkafy W, Cavero-Vanek S. The management of peripheral facial nerve palsy: "paresis" versus "paralysis" and sources of ambiguity in study designs. Otol Neurotol 2010;31:319–27.

5. Jowett N, Hadlock TA. Contemporary management of Bell's palsy. Facial Plastic Surgery 2015;31(2):93–102.

6. Rivas A, Boahene KD, Bravo HC, et al. A model for early prediction of facial nerve recovery after vestibular schwannoma surgery. Otol Neurotol 2011;32:826–33.

7. Anderson RL, Gordy DD. The tarsal strip procedure. Arch Ophthalmol 1979;97:2192–6.

8. Gillies H. Experiences with fascia lata grafts in the operative treatment of facial paralysis (section of otology and section of laryngology). Proc R Soc Med 1934;27:1372–82.

9. McLaughlin CR. Permanent facial paralysis: the role of surgical support. Lancet 1952;2:647–51.

10. Harii K, Ohmori K, Torii S. Free gracilis muscle transplantation, with microneurovascular anastomoses for the treatment of facial paralysis. A preliminary report. Plast Reconstr Surg 1976;57:133–43.

11. Harii K, Asato H, Yoshimura K, et al. One-stage transfer of the latissimus dorsi muscle for reanimation of a paralyzed face: a new alternative. Plast Reconstr Surg 1998;102:941–51.

12. Edgerton MT. Surgical correction of facial paralysis: a plea for better reconstructions. Ann Surg 1967;165:985–98.

13. Terzis JK, Kalantarian B. Microsurgical strategies in 74 patients for restoration of dynamic depressor muscle mechanism: a neglected target in facial reanimation. Plast Reconstr Surg 2000;105:1917–31 [discussion: 1932–4].

14. Watanabe Y, Sasaki R, Agawa K, et al. Bidirectional/double fascia grafting for simple and semidynamic reconstruction of lower lip deformity in facial paralysis. J Plast Reconstr Aesthet Surg 2015;68:321–8.

15. Wernick Robinson M, Baiungo J, Hohman M, et al. Facial rehabilitation. Operative Techniques in Otolaryngology-Head and Neck Surgery 2012;23:288–96.

16. House JW. Facial nerve grading systems. Laryngoscope 1983;93:1056–69.

17. House JW, Brackmann DE. Facial nerve grading system. Otolaryngol Head Neck Surg 1985;93:146–7.

18. Fisch U. Surgery for Bell's palsy. Arch Otolaryngol 1981;107:1–11.

19. Botman JW, Jongkees LB. The result of intratemporal treatment of facial palsy. Pract Otorhinolaryngol (Basel) 1955;17:80–100.

20. May M, Blumenthal F, Taylor FH. Bell's palsy: surgery based upon prognostic indicators and results. Laryngoscope 1981;91:2092–103.

21. Yanagihara N. On standardised documentation of facial palsy (author's transl). Nihon Jibiinkoka Gakkai kaiho 1977;80:799–805 [in Japanese].

22. Ross BG, Fradet G, Nedzelski JM. Development of a sensitive clinical facial grading system. Otolaryngol Head Neck Surg 1996;114:380–6.

23. Ross BR, Fradet G, Nedzelski JM. Development of a sensitive clinical facial grading system. Eur Arch Otorhinolaryngol 1994;S180–1.

24. Banks CA, Hadlock TA. Pediatric facial nerve rehabilitation. Facial Plast Surg Clin North Am 2014;22: 487–502.

25. Banks CA, Bhama PK, Park J, et al. Cliniciangraded electronic facial paralysis assessment: the eFACE. Plast Reconstr Surg, in print.

26. Bray D, Henstrom DK, Cheney ML, et al. Assessing outcomes in facial reanimation: evaluation and validation of the SMILE system for measuring lip excursion during smiling. Arch Facial Plast Surg 2010; 12:352–4.

27. Stewart MG, Witsell DL, Smith TL, et al. Development and validation of the Nasal Obstruction Symptom Evaluation (NOSE) scale. Otolaryngol Head Neck Surg 2004;130:157–63.

28. Lindsay RW, Smitson C, Edwards C, et al. Correction of the nasal base in the flaccidly paralyzed face: an orphaned problem in facial paralysis. Plast Reconstr Surg 2010;126:185e–6e.

29. Ware JE Jr, Sherbourne CD. The MOS 36-item short-form health survey (SF-36). I. Conceptual framework and item selection. Med Care 1992;30: 473–83.

30. VanSwearingen JM, Brach JS. The facial disability index: reliability and validity of a disability assessment instrument for disorders of the facial neuromuscular system. Phys Ther 1996;76:1288–98 [discussion: 98–300].

31. Bhama P, Bhrany AD. Ocular protection in facial paralysis. Curr Opin Otolaryngol Head Neck Surg 2013;21:353–7.

32. Gire A, Kwok A, Marx DP. PROSE treatment for lagophthalmos and exposure keratopathy. Ophthal Plast Reconstr Surg 2013;29:e38–40.

33. Weyns M, Koppen C, Tassignon MJ. Scleral contact lenses as an alternative to tarsorrhaphy for the long-term management of combined exposure and neurotrophic keratopathy. Cornea 2013;32: 359–61.

34. de Almeida JR, Guyatt GH, Sud S, et al. Management of Bell palsy: clinical practice guideline. CMAJ 2014;186:917–22.

35. Baugh RF, Basura GJ, Ishii LE, et al. Clinical practice guideline: Bell's palsy. Otolaryngol Head Neck Surg 2013;149:S1–27.

36. de Almeida JR, Al Khabori M, Guyatt GH, et al. Combined corticosteroid and antiviral treatment for Bell palsy: a systematic review and meta-analysis. JAMA 2009;302:985–93.

37. Sullivan FM, Swan IR, Donnan PT, et al. Early treatment with prednisolone or acyclovir in Bell's palsy. N Engl J Med 2007;357:1598–607.

38. De Diego JI, Prim MP, De Sarria MJ, et al. Idiopathic facial paralysis: a randomized, prospective, and controlled study using single-dose prednisone versus acyclovir three times daily. Laryngoscope 1998;108:573–5.

39. McAllister K, Walker D, Donnan PT, et al. Surgical interventions for the early management of Bell's palsy. Cochrane Database Syst Rev 2013;(10):CD007468.

40. Beutner KR, Friedman DJ, Forszpaniak C, et al. Valaciclovir compared with acyclovir for improved therapy for herpes zoster in immunocompetent adults. Antimicrob Agents Chemother 1995;39: 1546–53.

41. Murakami S, Hato N, Horiuchi J, et al. Treatment of Ramsay Hunt syndrome with acyclovir-prednisone: significance of early diagnosis and treatment. Ann Neurol 1997;41:353–7.

42. Coulson S, Croxson GR, Adams R, et al. Prognostic factors in herpes zoster oticus (Ramsay Hunt syndrome). Otol Neurotol 2011;32:1025–30.

43. Darrouzet V, Duclos JY, Liguoro D, et al. Management of facial paralysis resulting from temporal bone fractures: our experience in 115 cases. Otolaryngol Head Neck Surg 2001;125:77–84.

44. Kim J, Moon IS, Lee WS. Effect of delayed decompression after early steroid treatment on facial function of patients with facial paralysis. Acta Otolaryngol 2010;130:179–84.

45. Centers for Disease Control and Prevention (CDC). Lyme disease–United States, 2003-2005. MMWR Morb Mortal Wkly Rep 2007;56:573–6.

46. Wormser GP, Dattwyler RJ, Shapiro ED, et al. The clinical assessment, treatment, and prevention of Lyme disease, human granulocytic anaplasmosis, and babesiosis: clinical practice guidelines by the Infectious Diseases Society of America. Clin Infect Dis 2006;43:1089–134.

47. Kalish RA, Kaplan RF, Taylor E, et al. Evaluation of study patients with Lyme disease, 10-20-year follow-up. J Infect Dis 2001;183:453–60.

48. Clark JR, Carlson RD, Sasaki CT, et al. Facial paralysis in Lyme disease. Laryngoscope 1985;95: 1341–5.

49. Joseph EM, Sperling NM. Facial nerve paralysis in acute otitis media: cause and management revisited. Otolaryngol Head Neck Surg 1998;118: 694–6.

50. Redaelli de Zinis LO, Gamba P, Balzanelli C. Acute otitis media and facial nerve paralysis in adults. Otol Neurotol 2003;24:113–7.

51. Gantz BJ, Rubinstein JT, Gidley P, et al. Surgical management of Bell's palsy. Laryngoscope 1999; 109:1177–88.

52. May M, Klein SR, Taylor FH. Indications for surgery for Bell's palsy. Am J Otol 1984;5:503–12.

53. May M, Klein SR, Taylor FH. Idiopathic (Bell's) facial palsy: natural history defies steroid or surgical treatment. Laryngoscope 1985;95:406–9.

54. Liu Y, Han J, Zhou X, et al. Surgical management of facial paralysis resulting from temporal bone fractures. Acta Otolaryngol 2014;134:656–60.

55. Hato N, Nota J, Hakuba N, et al. Facial nerve decompression surgery in patients with temporal bone trauma: analysis of 66 cases. J Trauma 2011;71:1789–92 [discussion: 1792–3].

56. Vrabec JT, Lin JW. Acute paralysis of the facial nerve. In: Johnson JT, Rosen CA, editors. Bailey's head and neck surgery: otolaryngology. 5th edition. Philadelphia: Wolters Kluwer Health/Lippincott Williams & Wilkins; 2014. p. 2503–18.

57. Nash JJ, Friedland DR, Boorsma KJ, et al. Management and outcomes of facial paralysis from intratemporal blunt trauma: a systematic review. Laryngoscope 2010;120:1397–404.

58. Peitersen E. The natural history of Bell's palsy. Am J Otol 1982;4:107–11.

59. Aydin MA, Mackinnon SE, Gu XM, et al. Force deficits in skeletal muscle after delayed reinnervation. Plast Reconstr Surg 2004;113:1712–8.

60. Ma J, Shen J, Garrett JP, et al. Gene expression of myogenic regulatory factors, nicotinic acetylcholine receptor subunits, and GAP-43 in skeletal muscle following denervation in a rat model. J Orthop Res 2007;25:1498–505.

61. Wu P, Chawla A, Spinner RJ, et al. Key changes in denervated muscles and their impact on regeneration and reinnervation. Neural Regen Res 2014;9: 1796–809.

62. Conley J. Hypoglossal crossover–122 cases. Trans Sect Otolaryngol Am Acad Ophthalmol Otolaryngol 1977;84:ORL-763–8.

63. Gavron JP, Clemis JD. Hypoglossal-facial nerve anastomosis: a review of forty cases caused by facial nerve injuries in the posterior fossa. Laryngoscope 1984;94:1447–50.

64. Kunihiro T, Kanzaki J, Yoshihara S, et al. Hypoglossal-facial nerve anastomosis after acoustic neuroma resection: influence of the time anastomosis on recovery of facial movement. ORL J Otorhinolaryngol Relat Spec 1996;58:32–5.

65. Luff AR. Age-associated changes in the innervation of muscle fibers and changes in the mechanical properties of motor units. Ann N Y Acad Sci 1998; 854:92–101.

66. Pollin MM, McHanwell S, Slater CR. The effect of age on motor neurone death following axotomy in the mouse. Development 1991;112:83–9.

67. Vaughan DW. Effects of advancing age on peripheral nerve regeneration. J Comp Neurol 1992;323: 219–37.

68. Kovacic U, Sketelj J, Bajrovic FF. Chapter 26: Age-related differences in the reinnervation after peripheral nerve injury. Int Rev Neurobiol 2009; 87:465–82.

69. McGuirt WF, McCabe BF. Effect of radiation therapy on facial nerve cable autografts. Laryngoscope 1977;87:415–28.

70. McGuirt WF, Welling DB, McCabe BF. Facial nerve function following irradiated cable grafts. Laryngoscope 1989;99:27–34.

71. Brown PD, Eshleman JS, Foote RL, et al. An analysis of facial nerve function in irradiated and unirradiated facial nerve grafts. Int J Radiat Oncol Biol Phys 2000;48:737–43.

72. Reddy PG, Arden RL, Mathog RH. Facial nerve rehabilitation after radical parotidectomy. Laryngoscope 1999;109:894–9.

73. Maeda T, Hori S, Sasaki S, et al. Effects of tension at the site of coaptation on recovery of sciatic nerve function after neurorrhaphy: evaluation by walking-track measurement, electrophysiology, histomorphometry, and electron probe X-ray microanalysis. Microsurgery 1999;19:200–7.

74. Zhang F, Inserra M, Richards L, et al. Quantification of nerve tension after nerve repair: correlations with nerve defects and nerve regeneration. J Reconstr Microsurg 2001;17:445–51.

75. Sunderland IR, Brenner MJ, Singham J, et al. Effect of tension on nerve regeneration in rat sciatic nerve transection model. Ann Plast Surg 2004;53:382–7.

76. Yi C, Dahlin LB. Impaired nerve regeneration and Schwann cell activation after repair with tension. Neuroreport 2010;21:958–62.

77. Miyamoto Y. Experimental study of results of nerve suture under tension vs. nerve grafting. Plast Reconstr Surg 1979;64:540–9.

78. Bora FW Jr, Richardson S, Black J. The biomechanical responses to tension in a peripheral nerve. J Hand Surg Am 1980;5:21–5.

79. Stromberg BV, Vlastou C, Earle AS. Effect of nerve graft polarity on nerve regeneration and function. J Hand Surg Am 1979;4:444–5.

80. Sotereanos DG, Seaber AV, Urbaniak JR, et al. Reversing nerve-graft polarity in a rat model: the effect on function. J Reconstr Microsurg 1992;8:303–7.

81. Nakatsuka H, Takamatsu K, Koshimune M, et al. Experimental study of polarity in reversing cable nerve grafts. J Reconstr Microsurg 2002;18:509–15.

82. Ansselin AD, Davey DF. Axonal regeneration through peripheral nerve grafts: the effect of

proximo-distal orientation. Microsurgery 1988;9:
103–13.

83. Cabaud HE, Rodkey WG, McCarroll HR Jr, et al. Epineurial and perineurial fascicular nerve repairs: a critical comparison. J Hand Surg Am 1976;1: 131–7.

84. Orgel MG, Terzis JK. Epineurial vs. perineurial repair. Plast Reconstr Surg 1977;60:80–91.

85. Murray JA, Willins M, Mountain RE. A comparison of epineurial and perineurial sutures for the repair of a divided rat sciatic nerve. Clin Otolaryngol Allied Sci 1994;19:95–7.

86. Bratton BR, Kline DG, Coleman W, et al. Experimental interfascicular nerve grafting. J Neurosurg 1979;51:323–32.

87. Levinthal R, Brown WJ, Rand RW. Comparison of fascicular, interfascicular and epineural suture techniques in the repair of simple nerve lacerations. J Neurosurg 1977;47:744–50.

88. Rodkey WG, Cabaud HE, McCarroll HR Jr. Neurorrhaphy after loss of a nerve segment: comparison of epineurial suture under tension versus multiple nerve grafts. J Hand Surg Am 1980;5:366–71.

89. Hudson AR, Hunter D, Kline DG, et al. Histological studies of experimental interfascicular graft repairs. J Neurosurg 1979;51:333–40.

90. Knox CJ, Hohman MH, Kleiss IJ, et al. Facial nerve repair: fibrin adhesive coaptation versus epineurial suture repair in a rodent model. Laryngoscope 2013;123:1618–21.

91. Rafijah G, Bowen AJ, Dolores C, et al. The effects of adjuvant fibrin sealant on the surgical repair of segmental nerve defects in an animal model. J Hand Surg Am 2013;38:847–55.

92. Boedts D. A comparative experimental study on nerve repair. Arch Otorhinolaryngol 1987;244:1–6.

93. Menovsky T, Beek JF. Laser, fibrin glue, or suture repair of peripheral nerves: a comparative functional, histological, and morphometric study in the rat sciatic nerve. J Neurosurg 2001;95:694–9.

94. Tetik C, Ozer K, Ayhan S, et al. Conventional versus epineural sleeve neurorrhaphy technique: functional and histomorphometric analysis. Ann Plast Surg 2002;49:397–403.

95. Martins RS, Siqueira MG, Da Silva CF, et al. Overall assessment of regeneration in peripheral nerve lesion repair using fibrin glue, suture, or a combination of the 2 techniques in a rat model. Which is the ideal choice? Surg Neurol 2005;64(Suppl 1). p. S1: 10–6. [discussion: S1:6].

96. Martins RS, Siqueira MG, Silva CF, et al. Electrophysiologic assessment of regeneration in rat sciatic nerve repair using suture, fibrin glue or a combination of both techniques. Arq Neuropsiquiatr 2005;63:601–4.

97. Ornelas L, Padilla L, Di Silvio M, et al. Fibrin glue: an alternative technique for nerve coaptation–Part I.

Wave amplitude, conduction velocity, and plantar-length factors. J Reconstr Microsurg 2006;22: 119–22.

98. Ornelas L, Padilla L, Di Silvio M, et al. Fibrin glue: an alternative technique for nerve coaptation–Part II. Nerve regeneration and histomorphometric assessment. J Reconstr Microsurg 2006; 22:123–8.

99. Sameem M, Wood TJ, Bain JR. A systematic review on the use of fibrin glue for peripheral nerve repair. Plast Reconstr Surg 2011;127:2381–90.

100. Povlsen B. A new fibrin seal in primary repair of peripheral nerves. J Hand Surg Br 1994;19:43–7.

101. Smahel J, Meyer VE, Bachem U. Glueing of peripheral nerves with fibrin: experimental studies. J Reconstr Microsurg 1987;3:211–20.

102. Suri A, Mehta VS, Sarkar C. Microneural anastomosis with fibrin glue: an experimental study. Neurol India 2002;50:23–6.

103. Medders G, Mattox DE, Lyles A. Effects of fibrin glue on rat facial nerve regeneration. Otolaryngol Head Neck Surg 1989;100:106–9.

104. Moy OJ, Peimer CA, Koniuch MP, et al. Fibrin seal adhesive versus nonabsorbable microsuture in peripheral nerve repair. J Hand Surg Am 1988;13: 273–8.

105. Maragh H, Meyer BS, Davenport D, et al. Morphofunctional evaluation of fibrin glue versus microsuture nerve repairs. J Reconstr Microsurg 1990;6: 331–7.

106. Junior ED, Valmaseda-Castellon E, Gay-Escoda C. Facial nerve repair with epineural suture and anastomosis using fibrin adhesive: an experimental study in the rabbit. J Oral Maxillofac Surg 2004; 62:1524–9.

107. Egloff DV, Narakas A. Nerve anastomoses with human fibrin. Preliminary clinical report (56 cases). Ann Chir Main 1983;2:101–15.

108. Bozorg Grayeli A, Mosnier I, Julien N, et al. Long-term functional outcome in facial nerve graft by fibrin glue in the temporal bone and cerebellopontine angle. Eur Arch Otorhinolaryngol 2005;262: 404–7.

109. Sterkers O, Becherel P, Sterkers JM. Repair of the facial nerve exclusively by fibrin glue. 56 cases. Ann Otolaryngol Chir Cervicofac 1989;106:176–81 [in French].

110. Wieken K, Angioi-Duprez K, Lim A, et al. Nerve anastomosis with glue: comparative histologic study of fibrin and cyanoacrylate glue. J Reconstr Microsurg 2003;19:17–20.

111. Teixeira LJ, Valbuza JS, Prado GF. Physical therapy for Bell's palsy (idiopathic facial paralysis). Cochrane Database Syst Rev 2011;(12): CD006283.

112. Beurskens CH, Heymans PG. Positive effects of mime therapy on sequelae of facial paralysis: stiffness, lip

mobility, and social and physical aspects of facial disability. Otol Neurotol 2003;24:677–81.

113. Beurskens CH, Heymans PG, Oostendorp RA. Stability of benefits of mime therapy in sequelae of facial nerve paresis during a 1-year period. Otol Neurotol 2006;27:1037–42.

114. Pourmomeny AA, Zadmehre H, Mirshamsi M, et al. Prevention of synkinesis by biofeedback therapy: a randomized clinical trial. Otol Neurotol 2014;35:739–42.

115. Nicastri M, Mancini P, De Seta D, et al. Efficacy of early physical therapy in severe Bell's palsy: a randomized controlled trial. Neurorehabil Neural Repair 2013;27:542–51.

116. Borodic G, Bartley M, Slattery W, et al. Botulinum toxin for aberrant facial nerve regeneration: double-blind, placebo-controlled trial using subjective endpoints. Plast Reconstr Surg 2005;116:36–43.

117. Chen CK, Tang YB. Myectomy and botulinum toxin for paralysis of the marginal mandibular branch of the facial nerve: a series of 76 cases. Plast Reconstr Surg 2007;120:1859–64.

118. Krohel GB, Cipollo CL, Gaddipati K. Contralateral botulinum injections improve drinking ability and facial symmetry in patients with facial paralysis. Am J Ophthalmol 2005;139:540.

119. Clark RP, Berris CE. Botulinum toxin: a treatment for facial asymmetry caused by facial nerve paralysis. Plast Reconstr Surg 1989;84:353–5.

120. Takushima A, Harii K, Sugawara Y, et al. Anthropometric measurements of the endoscopic eyebrow lift in the treatment of facial paralysis. Plast Reconstr Surg 2003;111:2157–65.

121. Ueda K, Harii K, Yamada A. Long-term follow-up study of browlift for treatment of facial paralysis. Ann Plast Surg 1994;32:166–70.

122. Hohman MH, Silver AL, Henstrom DK, et al. The "power" brow lift: efficient correction of the paralyzed brow. ISRN Plastic Surgery 2013;2013:4.

123. Pakarinen M, Tervo T, Tarkkanen A. Tarsorraphy in the treatment of persistent corneal lesions. Acta Ophthalmol Suppl 1987;182:69–73.

124. Cosar CB, Cohen EJ, Rapuano CJ, et al. Tarsorrhaphy: clinical experience from a cornea practice. Cornea 2001;20:787–91.

125. May M. Gold weight and wire spring implants as alternatives to tarsorrhaphy. Arch Otolaryngol Head Neck Surg 1987;113:656–60.

126. Levine RE, Shapiro JP. Reanimation of the paralyzed eyelid with the enhanced palpebral spring or the gold weight: modern replacements for tarsorrhaphy. Facial Plast Surg 2000;16:325–36.

127. Schrom T, Habermann A, Wernecke K, et al. Implantation of lid weights for therapy of lagophthalmos. Ophthalmologe 2005;102:1186–92 [in German].

128. Silver AL, Lindsay RW, Cheney ML, et al. Thin-profile platinum eyelid weighting: a superior option in the paralyzed eye. Plast Reconstr Surg 2009;123:1697–703.

129. Terzis JK, Kyere SA. Minitendon graft transfer for suspension of the paralyzed lower eyelid: our experience. Plast Reconstr Surg 2008;121:1206–16.

130. Golio D, De Martelaere S, Anderson J, et al. Outcomes of periocular reconstruction for facial nerve paralysis in cancer patients. Plast Reconstr Surg 2007;119:1233–7.

131. Olver JM. Surgical tips on the lateral tarsal strip. Eye 1998;12(Pt 6):1007–12.

132. Hohman MH, Lee LN, Hadlock TA. Two-step highly selective neurectomy for refractory periocular synkinesis. Laryngoscope 2013;123:1385–8.

133. Bhama PK, Park JG, Shanley K, et al. Refinements in nasolabial fold reconstruction for facial paralysis. Laryngoscope 2014;124:2687–92.

134. Lindsay RW, Bhama P, Hohman M, et al. Prospective evaluation of quality-of-life improvement after correction of the alar base in the flaccidly paralyzed face. JAMA Facial Plast Surg 2015;17(2):108–12.

135. Hadlock TA, Greenfield LJ, Wernick-Robinson M, et al. Multimodality approach to management of the paralyzed face. Laryngoscope 2006;116:1385–9.

136. Constantinides M, Galli SK, Miller PJ. Complications of static facial suspensions with expanded polytetrafluoroethylene (ePTFE). Laryngoscope 2001;111:2114–21.

137. Hadlock TA, Malo JS, Cheney ML, et al. Free gracilis transfer for smile in children: the Massachusetts Eye and Ear Infirmary Experience in excursion and quality-of-life changes. Arch Facial Plast Surg 2011;13:190–4.

138. Bhama PK, Weinberg JS, Lindsay RW, et al. Objective outcomes analysis following microvascular gracilis transfer for facial reanimation: a review of 10 years' experience. JAMA Facial Plast Surg 2014;16:85–92.

139. Cuccia G, Shelley O, d'Alcontres FS, et al. A comparison of temporalis transfer and free latissimus dorsi transfer in lower facial reanimation following unilateral longstanding facial palsy. Ann Plast Surg 2005;54:66–70.

140. Hussain G, Manktelow RT, Tomat LR. Depressor labii inferioris resection: an effective treatment for marginal mandibular nerve paralysis. Br J Plast Surg 2004;57:502–10.

141. Rubin LR. The anatomy of a smile: its importance in the treatment of facial paralysis. Plast Reconstr Surg 1974;53:384–7.

142. Henstrom DK, Malo JS, Cheney ML, et al. Platysmectomy: an effective intervention for facial synkinesis and hypertonicity. Arch Facial Plast Surg 2011;13:239–43.

143. Sachs ME, Conley J. Functional and aesthetic consequences of total platysma resection. Arch Otolaryngol 1984;110:448–9.

144. Wollheim FA, Wollheim FA. Acute and long-term complications of corticosteroid pulse therapy. Scand J Rheumatol 1984;13:27–32.

145. McKee MD, Waddell JP, Kudo PA, et al. Osteonecrosis of the femoral head in men following short-course corticosteroid therapy: a report of 15 cases. CMAJ 2001;164:205–6.

Evidence-Based Facial Fracture Management

Timothy D. Doerr, MD, FACS

KEYWORDS

- Facial fractures • Trauma • Evidence-based • Surgery • Mandible • Nasal

KEY POINTS

- The facial trauma literature primarily consists of lower-level evidence, including retrospective case series and case reports.
- There is strong clinical evidence from meta-analysis to guide antibiotic use in facial trauma.
- There is solid clinical evidence from meta-analysis of clinical trials supporting the use of general anesthesia for closed nasal reduction.
- There is no consensus from the literature on the best method of treating mandible fractures.
- Systematic review of the literature suggests improved patient outcomes with open reduction for displaced fractures of the mandibular condyle.

INTRODUCTION

The demand for safe, cost-effective health care is increasing from the public, physicians, and third-party payers. Evidence-based practice is becoming an essential component of twenty-first century medicine and, increasingly, doctors must justify their work based on clinical effectiveness and cost. Physicians are being asked to show, using higher level clinical research, the clinical benefits of accepted treatments. However, many of these treatments developed through technical advances or surgical pioneering and were not vetted through the rigorous process of clinical trials.

Facial fracture management, like most aspects of facial plastic and reconstructive surgery, has evolved through the collective experiences of its surgeons. The current surgical trends and techniques have been shaped through advances in diagnostics, instrumentation, and hardware. In facial trauma, most current practices did not result from rigorous randomized clinical trials (RCTs). Instead, surgeons adopted new techniques and approaches when they believed them to be better than what had been done. There certainly was no requirement to prove the superiority of a new technique or instrument before adopting it. Innovators were not compelled to prove what they thought was inherently obvious.

It is not surprising that the literature concerning facial fracture treatment is limited both in its quality and level of evidence. The predominant article types are retrospective case series and non-randomized trials. There is a scarcity of RCTs in all of facial plastic surgery; however, it is very glaring in facial trauma. This is not surprising given the obstacles inherent in conducting clinical studies in fracture treatment. Cost, ethical constraints, and subject recruitment all deter randomized studies. There are also challenges in conducting surgical trials given the significant variability in facial fractures, the range of surgical procedures to address the injuries, and the skills of surgeons performing those operations.

Disclosures: AONA Faculty Member: receives honoraria and travel expenses for teaching educational courses. AO Foundation: Facial Trauma and Reconstructive Surgery Expert Group; receives per diem and travel expenses to attend working meetings. Depuy Synthes: paid consultant, material development.
Department of Otolaryngology–Head and Neck Surgery, University of Rochester School of Medicine and Dentistry, 601 Elmwood, Box 629, Rochester, NY 14642, USA
E-mail address: timothy_doerr@urmc.rochester.edu

Facial Plast Surg Clin N Am 23 (2015) 335–345
http://dx.doi.org/10.1016/j.fsc.2015.04.006
1064-7406/15/$ – see front matter © 2015 Elsevier Inc. All rights reserved.

Recognizing that facial fracture management has evolved over decades mostly devoid of any evidence-based research, and further recognizing the persistent challenges in conducting quality studies, it is easy to view evidenced-based facial fracture care as unattainable. However, some recent studies in facial fracture treatment have included higher level randomized trials as well as organized meta-analysis. As specialists, facial plastic surgeons must continue to adapt evidence-based approaches to both clinical practice and research. Doing so validates what we are doing well and highlights areas needing improvement. Both the public and organized medicine demands this research and our specialty needs to provide it.

This article reviews relevant issues in facial fracture management, emphasizing the evidence-based methodology. It highlights the few areas of facial trauma in which randomized studies and meta-analysis are available. It also points out the many other areas for which the evidenced-based literature is poor or altogether absent. Finally, the article examines the future of facial trauma care in which clinical registries and health databases may be better able to answer clinical questions too complex to be addressed by clinical trials.

ANTIBIOTICS AND FACIAL FRACTURES

The role of antibiotics in facial fracture treatment remains unsettled and controversial. With injuries varying widely in fracture location, severity, and wound contamination, the clinical benefits of antibiotics use is not easily determined. The literature on this topic is complex and at times conflicting. With the increasing rates of antibiotic resistance and calls for an evidence-based approach to patient care, clarifying the role for antibiotic use in facial trauma is important. The literature has tried to distinguish between antibiotic use in mandible fractures and antibiotics with other facial fractures, including those isolated mandibular condyle fractures. Surgeons agree on the need for antibiotics with infected wounds and most routinely administer antibiotics in the perioperative setting. The literature supporting preoperative antibiotic use is not clear-cut and the use of postoperative antibiotics is even more controversial.

In 2006, Andreasen and colleagues[1] conducted a systematic review to identify the potential benefit of prophylactic antibiotics in the maxillofacial fractures. The reviewers sought to address 3 important questions: does antibiotic prophylaxis decrease infections in jaw fracture treatment, are there situations when antibiotic prophylaxis is not indicated, and which is the antibiotic prescription

of choice? They identified 4 RCTs that met the search criteria. Collectively, the studies showed a 3-fold decrease in infection rates for mandibular fractures in the antibiotic-treated groups compared with the no-antibiotic control groups. The review identified a wide variety of antibiotics that seemed to have a uniform effect in reducing infections. The review further noted that the reduction in infections was seen regardless of antibiotic duration. However, there was no benefit to giving postoperative antibiotics beyond 24 to 48 hours. Only 1 of the 4 studies actually looked at antibiotics in facial fractures other than the mandible. This trial found no infections with repairs of maxillary, zygoma, or condyle fractures. The reviewers concluded that prophylactic antibiotics are beneficial in the treatment of mandible fractures but, because of a low risk of postoperative infection, prophylactic antibiotics were not indicated for other facial fracture sites.

In 2011, Kyzas[2] published another comprehensive systematic review of antibiotics and mandible fractures with slightly different conclusions. Challenging the notion that antibiotic use in mandible fractures was mandatory, and spurred by the weak literature previously highlighted, Kyzas sought to more clearly define the role for antibiotics. This review included 9 randomized trials and 22 nonrandomized retrospective case series. He found the literature to be of poor quality with variable data that prohibited making any quantitative assessments. The reviewed studies had infection rates ranging from 4.5% to 62% without antibiotics and from 1.9% to 29.4% with antibiotics. He concluded that the support for prophylactic antibiotic use was limited and of weak quality. Based on his analysis, any recommendation for routine antibiotic use was weak and not reliably supported by the literature.

To determine the benefit of postoperative antibiotics after mandible fracture repair, Miles and colleagues[3] conducted a prospective RCT. All subjects received preoperative and intraoperative antibiotics. Eighty-one subjects also received postoperative antibiotics and 100 had no postoperative antibiotics. There were no differences in postoperative infection rates. There were infections in 8 out of 81 subjects who received postoperative antibiotics and 14 out of 100 who did not receive postoperative antibiotics. The investigators were unable to show a benefit of using postoperative antibiotics for mandible fracture repair.

A 2014 systematic review by Shridharani and colleagues[4] also looked at the potential benefit of antibiotics after mandible fracture repair. Their review found 73 potential articles with only 5 meeting defined criteria. They noted that, although several studies addressed the antibiotic question, there was wide variability in antibiotics, subjects, and treatment protocols. They suggested there was a trend toward not needing antibiotics beyond 24 hours after fracture repair. They cautioned that this lower degree of evidence with its limited number of level 1 studies did not provide a gold standard for management. To highlight what are clear differences between actual clinical practice and the prevailing literature, the reviewers also presented results from a surgeon survey in which more than 50% of respondents routinely used postoperative antibiotics despite the lack of supporting evidence.

The literature examining the role of antibiotic prophylaxis in nonmandibular facial fractures is even sparser. In a multi-institutional prospective cohort study, Knepil and Loukota[5] studied prophylactic antibiotics in 134 subjects who had surgery for zygoma fractures. They found a postoperative infection rate of only 1.5%, which was seen only after transoral surgical approach.

Summarizing the available literature, Morris and Kellman[6] recommend that antibiotics be given for mandible fractures only from injury until completion of the perioperative course but not postoperatively. There are insufficient data to assess prophylactic antibiotics in nonmandible fractures and isolated condyle fractures but evidence that did exist suggested no benefit to postoperative antibiotics (**Table 1**).

Having highlighted the indications for antibiotics in facial fracture repair, comment on the role of antibiotics in skull base trauma is necessary. There is controversy about whether antibiotics should be routinely given to patients with skull base fractures in an effort to prevent infectious complications, including meningitis. Previous publications have both called for and recommended against this practice.[7,8] In 2011, Ratilal and colleagues[9] published a Cochrane review of RCTs as well as non-RCTS concerning antibiotics and skull base

fracture. The review identified 5 RCTs involving 208 subjects. Analysis showed no reduction in meningitis rates, overall mortality, meningitis-related mortality, and the need for surgery from cerebrospinal fluid leak in subjects receiving prophylactic antibiotics. No complications from antibiotic use were seen; however, 1 study did find a change in the microbial flora toward organisms more likely to be resistant to antibiotics. In addition, the review examined 17 nonrandomized studies, which included more than 2100 subjects. The analysis produced results in line with those seen in the randomized data. Most of studies lacked sufficient details on methodology, which limited their quality. The conclusion of this analysis was that there was insufficient evidence for prophylactic antibiotic use in patients with skull base fractures with or without a cerebrospinal fluid leak. Until better evidence becomes available, the routine use of antibiotics in these cases should be avoided.

NASAL FRACTURES

No facial injury is more common than the nasal fracture. Despite a frequency of injury that should lend to clinical investigation, there are only a handful of randomized trials examining nasal trauma management. Although closed reduction for a nasal fracture is common practice and, in some locations, the standard of care, the efficacy of this procedure is still debated. Although many surgeons advocate for closed nasal reduction, others encourage more extensive open techniques to address nasal injuries. Extensive-fracture dislocation of the nasal bone and septum, dramatic deviation of the nasal pyramid, dislocation or open fractures of the septum, and persistent deformity after an attempt at closed reduction are directing surgeons to an consider an open approach.[10] Some recent publications have even advocated for a more formal rhinoplasty approach with nearly

Table 1			
Role for antibiotics in facial fracture treatment			
	Antibiotics Before Surgery	Perioperative Antibiotics (within 2 h of surgery)	Prophylactic Antibiotics After Surgery
Mandible fractures (not isolated condyle)	Yes	Yes	No benefit to antibiotics beyond 24–48 h
Isolated mandibular condyle fractures	No benefit	Yes	No benefit
Midface and frontal sinus fracture	No benefit	Yes	No benefit
Skull base fractures	No role for prophylactic antibiotics with or without cerebrospinal fluid leak Role for antibiotics with skull base fracture repair not defined		

all of these injuries.[11] Despite the ongoing controversy, no prospective RCT has been conducted to directly compare open and closed techniques and help answer this clinical question.

In assessing the efficacy of nasal injury treatment, a 2002 publication by Staffel[12] deserves comment. He reported on the effectiveness of closed nasal reduction by reviewing several studies in the literature and proposing a treatment algorithm to improve outcomes. He also highlighted a dichotomy between high patient satisfaction with the clinical outcomes (79%) and the low surgeon satisfaction (37%) with those same results. This demonstrates that patient and surgeon expectations can be quite different and suggests that, if patient satisfaction is a primary goal of treatment, closed nasal reduction is likely the appropriate initial approach.

There is also no consensus on the best method of anesthesia for reducing a nasal fracture. Previous studies have shown that general anesthesia, sedation, and local anesthesia can all be effective and are well tolerated by subjects undergoing nasal reduction.[13–15] Anesthesia selection is often guided by surgeon preference, operating room availability, and hospital protocol. Advocates for general anesthesia have suggested that reduction can be performed with better outcomes and less pain,[14,15] whereas others showed equivalent outcomes at a lower cost using local anesthesia[13]

To address choice of anesthesia for closed nasal reduction Al-Moraissi and Ellis[16] conducted a systematic review of the literature with a meta-analysis. The review identified 8 studies with 846 subjects. Of these studies, 3 were RCTs, 2 were clinical cohort studies, and 3 were retrospective series. The analysis showed subject satisfaction with anesthesia and subject satisfaction with nasal function were both slightly higher, but not statistically higher, under general anesthesia. The subject satisfaction with nasal appearance was statistically higher with general anesthesia (**Table 2**). These subjects were also less likely to later require a secondary nasal procedure. These results support improved outcomes when nasal reduction is performed under general anesthesia; however,

this must be balanced against other factors, including procedure cost and convenience. Regardless of the anesthesia use in nasal reduction, other clinical factors, including septal and nasal tip deviation, are predictors of a persistent deformity and must be considered in selecting the method of treatment.

MANDIBLE FRACTURES

Mandible fractures are common fractures that encompass a variety of different injuries with an extensive range of treatment options. This diverse group of fractures can be treated with either open or closed reduction, followed by external or internal fixation, or both. Given the variety of fractures and the plethora of treatment options, it is not surprising that there is little consensus about which treatment is best for a specific fracture pattern.

Advancements in plating systems and a better understanding of the biomechanics of the mandible have led to a gradual evolution in fracture management. Closed reduction with mandibular-maxillary fixation (MMF) is increasingly being replaced by open approaches with application of various fixation hardware. As with most of facial trauma, there is limited high-level evidence to support such a clinical change. Most of the thousands of publications on mandible fracture repair are retrospective studies of suboptimal quality. Only recently have quality randomized trials looking at various aspects of mandible fracture repair appeared in the literature. These RCTs have examined many different variables, including the use of single miniplates, locking plates, 3-dimensional plates, resorbable plates, and lag screws to treat adult mandible fractures.

Angle Fractures

Patients sustaining mandible trauma usually present with defined anatomic fracture patterns. Each anatomic fracture pattern offers several options for repair with internal fixation. The presence of third molars and thin cortices of bone make the mandibular angle among the most common sites of fracture. The fractures of the angle have been

---

Table 2
Anesthesia and clinical outcomes in nasal fracture closed reduction

	Patient Satisfaction with Anesthesia	Patient Satisfaction with Nasal Function	Patient Satisfaction with Nasal Appearance
General anesthesia	Slightly higher	Slightly higher	Significantly higher
Local anesthesia	Slightly lower	Slightly lower	Significantly lower

Adapted from Al-Moraissi EA, Ellis E. Local versus general anesthesia for the management of nasal bone fractures: a systematic review and meta-analysis. J Oral Maxillofac Surg 2015;73(4):606–15; with permission.

investigated with several RCTs (**Table 3**) attempting to determine the ideal method of fixation. Danda[17] conducted 1 such trial by comparing postoperative complications between angle fractures repaired with a standard Champy plate and fractures repaired with a Champy plate plus a second plate on lateral aspect of the mandible. In this study, with 27 subjects in each group, there was no difference in complication rates. He concluded that there is no benefit to using a second plate for noncomminuted angle fractures. Siddiqui and colleagues[18] also compared plating requirements for angle fractures. This RCT again compared using 1 miniplate (n = 36) to using 2 miniplates (n = 26) for noncomminuted angle fractures. There was no difference in total morbidity or complications between the techniques. The investigators concluded that 2 miniplates offered no additional benefit and increased costs.

In a larger RCT found in the facial fracture literature, Laverick and colleagues[19] compared angle fractures repaired with a traditional Champy plate along the oblique ridge with repairs using a laterally placed plate with a transbuccal approach and percutaneous trocar. In this study of 261 fractures, the transbuccal lateral plate had a much lower postoperative infection rate (5%) than those placed along the oblique ridge (20%). The lateral plates were also far less likely to need removal for infection. The results showed that transbuccal lateral plating did not require longer operative times and was associated with fewer complications. The investigators recommend using this technique for all angle fractures for which a Champy plate would have otherwise been used.

Sugar and colleagues[20] studied 140 consecutive subjects undergoing repair of mandibular angle fractures. They compared complications with standard intraoral plating along the oblique ridge with intraoral plus transbuccal plating along the lateral boarder. The study found, based on the measured outcomes of plate removal and infection requiring further surgery, that the combined transbuccal-oral procedure was safer and more effective than the standard intraoral technique. The investigators also showed, using a surgeon survey, that it was overwhelmingly preferred by the surgeons who performed both procedures.

Despite the appearance of these randomized trials in the recent literature, proving the superiority of any particular plating technique will continue to be a challenge to surgeons. These referenced randomized trials were mostly of small sample size and reported several outcome variables in a nonstandardized manner. The findings from these studies were in some cases conflicting. Until larger, better-designed, and more standardized clinical trials are conducted, surgeons must use caution when interpreting this literature and applying it to patient care.

Even when there is agreement on the fixation for a particular type of fracture, there is a wide range of opinions about the need for postoperative MMF. The duration of MMF is influenced by many clinical factors, including fracture location, fracture severity, and anticipated patient compliance. There is only limited lower level evidence to determine an optimal length of MMF. Recently, Adeyemi and colleagues[21] conducted an RCT comparing the standard 4 to 6 weeks of MMF with a treatment group receiving only 2 weeks. The investigators found that both groups healed their fractures but recovery of full mouth opening was more rapid with a shorter period of MMF. In another study addressing the duration of MMF, Kaplan and colleagues[22] compared mandible

Table 3
Mandibular angle fracture repair randomized controlled trials

Study	Question	Result	Conclusion
Danda,[17] 2010	1 vs 2 miniplates for noncomminuted fracture	No difference in complication	No benefit to second plate
Siddiqui et al,[18] 2007	1 vs 2 miniplates for noncomminuted fracture	No differences in total morbidity or complications	No benefit and increased cost with second plate
Laverick et al,[19] 2012	Traditional Champy plate vs lateral plate via transbuccal	Much lower complications with lateral plate	Lateral plate favored over Champy
Sugar et al,[20] 2009	Traditional Champy plate vs lateral via transbuccal	Fewer complications with lateral plate	Lateral plate favored over Champy and preferred by surgeons

Data from Refs.[17–20]

fractures repaired with miniplates plus 2 weeks of postoperative MMF with fractures repaired with no postoperative MMF. They found no differences between the groups in terms of weight loss, trismus, dental hygiene, or wound complications. These studies suggest that in the appropriate fractures, a brief period of MMF or no MMF does not seem to negatively affect outcomes and will improve patient satisfaction.

Looking to identify best practice for the management of fractures of the mandible, Nasser and colleagues[23] conducted a 2013 Cochrane review. The reviewers systematically assessed the management of adult mandibular fractures not involving the condyle. They identified 12 studies that met their inclusion criteria, with half of these studies having a high risk of bias and half having an unclear risk of bias. Not surprisingly, the studies were very different in design and included comparisons of many different surgical approaches, fixation techniques, and postoperative protocols. The studies also differed widely in terms of endpoints, with patient-oriented outcomes largely ignored and postoperative pain scores inadequately reported. This Cochrane review found only 1 or 2 studies all of small sample size conducted for each comparison or outcome. Thus, a pooled analysis was possible in only a couple of areas. From these data, no difference in postoperative infection was seen using either 1 or 2 miniplates to repair an angle fracture. This review otherwise failed to identify the effectiveness of any single treatment approach for mandible fractures without condylar involvement. The review investigators thought that the absence of high-quality evidence was due to the clinical diversity of subjects along with the lack of consistent assessment tools and standardized outcome measures. The review concluded that, until high-level evidence is available, treatment of mandible fractures should be based on surgeon experience and patient circumstances.

With the development of resorbable plating systems there has also been enthusiasm for the use of these systems to fix mandible fractures. In a Cochrane review, Dorri and colleagues[24] attempted to compare mandible fracture repairs with traditional titanium plates with those repaired with a resorbable plate. This systematic review was unable to identify any eligible studies for comparison. The review was able to identify 2 ongoing studies that were halted because of increased complications. The investigators concluded that, in the absence of any reliable high-level evidence, surgeons should rely on clinical experience. Based on the aborted trials, it does not seem that resorbable plates were as effective as titanium plates for the

mandible. In a clinical trial published after this review, Ahmed and colleagues[25] directly compared, in a randomized fashion, fractures repaired with titanium or resorbable plates. With at least 34 subjects in each group, the investigators noted increased implant failure in the resorbable group with more screw and plate breakage during placement. Conversely, more plate removals were required in the titanium group. These results further supplement the conclusions drawn by Dorri and colleagues.[24] Given the technical difficulties with resorbable plating and the increased costs of these fixation systems for mandible fractures, these are not supported by the current literature.

Condylar and Subcondylar Fractures

No area of facial fracture management generates more controversy than the treatment of condylar neck and subcondylar fractures. There are several techniques to manage these fractures. Some surgeons advocate for conservative treatment with MMF, whereas others encourage open reduction and internal fixation (ORIF). Those favoring conservative treatment maintain that patients gain an equivalent functional status without the risks of infection, scar, or facial nerve injury that can be associated with open techniques. Supporters of an open approach claim there is earlier return to function and less malocclusion when patients are treated with ORIF.

Several recent trials suggest improved outcomes with open repair of condylar fractures. In 2006, Eckelt and colleaues[26] presented a multi-institutional prospective RCT comparing open operative with conservative treatment of displaced condylar fractures. Eighty-eight subjects were randomized resulting in 66 subjects with 79 fractures. All fractures were displaced with either excessive angulation or more than 2 mm shortening of the vertical ramus. At 6 weeks and 6 months after treatment, the investigators found correct anatomic positioning significantly more often in the open group. They also saw significant difference in function along with less pain after an open approach. The study concluded that, although both groups gained acceptable occlusion results, open treatment was superior to all other studied outcomes.

In 2010, Singh and colleagues[27] looked at 40 subjects with displaced fractures of the condyle; again, either excessively angulated or shortened by more than 2 mm. Subject function, occlusion, and radiograph parameters were compared 6 months after treatment. This study showed that anatomic reduction was more accurate and functional parameters superior in the open treatment group. However, this study showed difference in final occlusion. Although both groups gained an acceptable occlusion, the open treatment was better in all other measures, including pain.

In 2010, Danda and colleagues[28] studied displaced unilateral subcondylar and condylar neck fractures. This study found better radiographic reduction with an open repair but otherwise no differences in functional parameters. They thought that, although there were no ultimate differences in the functional parameters, a better radiographic result and earlier return to function supported treatment by ORIF. Finally, Kotrashetti and colleagues[29] used a retromandibular approach for ORIF of subcondylar fractures and compared this with closed reduction with MMF. In this small RCT, 12 subjects were treated by closed reduction and 10 subjects underwent ORIF. With follow-up at 3 and 6 months, these investigators showed that ORIF of displaced subcondylar fractures was better clinically and radiographically than fractures treated by closed techniques.

Proponents of an open approach argue that obtaining a good clinical result with closed management requires early mobilization and aggressive physiotherapy. Even then, they note that the condyle is not its normal position and there is universally diminished ramus height. These observations justify an open approach whenever there is significant overlap or angulation. Proponents of the open approach point to these recent studies supporting a better overall result with an acceptably low risk of soft tissue and nerve complications.

There have been a few attempts to define the best evidence concerning management of condyle fractures by conducting systematic reviews of the world literature. Nussbaum and colleagues[30] identified 13 potential studies in a meta-analysis but found most of the available data were poor quality that limited any meaningful analysis. In 2010, Sharif and colleagues[31] attempted a Cochrane systematic review of all RCTs concerning management of condyle fractures. After reviewing all potentially relevant articles, they found no studies that met their inclusion criteria. Several of the articles were excluded for deficiencies in randomization or loss of subjects to follow-up. As a result, no treatment recommendations were offered.

Liu and colleagues[32] conducted a more recent meta-analysis comparing open versus closed management of condyle fractures. From the literature, they identified 4 studies totaling 177 subjects. They found that subjects treated with open management had statistically better function, less pain, and less malocclusion. No difference was seen in maximum opening. Interestingly, this meta-analysis included studies that Sharif and

colleagues[31] rejected for deficiencies in the randomization process. The Liu and colleagues[32] meta-analysis concluded that, although both treatment methods can yield acceptable functional results, an ORIF was superior to closed treatment of moderately displaced subcondylar fractures (**Table 4**).

Although the debate over condyle fracture management is not yet settled, there is an increasing body of evidence showing improved results with ORIF. With the interest in ORIF, there has also been interest in using an endoscopic approach to access these fractures to minimize facial nerve injury and avoid a scar. There has been a single randomized study comparing endoscopic with open repair of condyle fractures.[33] The study involved 34 fractures treated endoscopically and 40 treated with a standard open technique. The study found longer operative times in the endoscopic group but equivalent function. In fractures in the open treatment group, facial nerve injury was not significantly increased and surgical scars were deemed cosmetically acceptable.

Orbital Fractures

The management of orbital fractures also creates considerable debate among the various specialists treating these injuries. There is much uncertainty about which patients need surgery and when. There are also divergent opinions about what approach and which of the many materials

Table 4
Comparison of clinical outcomes: open versus closed repair of moderately displaced unilateral subcondylar and condylar neck fractures

	Open Reduction	Closed Treatment
Occlusion	+	+
Maximum opening	+	+
Deviation with opening	—	+
Chronic pain	—	+
Radiographic reduction	++	—
Restoration of ramus height	++	—
Avoidance of facial nerve injury	—	+
Facial scar	+[a]	+
Patient satisfaction	+	—

+, indicating the relative benefit of each approach.
[a] With transoral endoscopic approach.

is optimal for repair of these fractures. There is some evidence gained through a meta-analysis of retrospective studies that eyelid complications are increased with subciliary approaches to the orbit compared with the transconjunctival approach.[34] There are certain orbital fractures for which the indication for prompt surgery is agreed. However, in most other instances the need for surgery is less clear. In deciding whether to repair an orbital fracture, the surgeon takes into account several factors, including vision, ocular motility, diplopia, and cosmesis. The clinician must decide which patients can safely be observed and repaired later if is still necessary. Important in this process is deciding whether motility is reduced by mechanical entrapment, swelling, or contused ocular muscles. These factors can influence patient outcomes.

In 2014, Dubois and colleagues[35] conducted a systematic review of the orbital trauma literature to identify any controlled clinical trials on posttraumatic orbital reconstruction with a focus on the timing, or delay, of surgery. From this review, a total of 17 studies with 1579 subjects with orbital injuries were identified. This included a single RCT of 21 subjects that compared nasal septal and conchal cartilage for orbital blowout repair. That study found repair before 4 weeks had a positive effect on postoperative enophthalmos. However, the timing of surgery was not randomized and it was unclear what factors influenced earlier interventions. In the only other prospective study, 24 subjects undergoing orbital fracture repair were followed for more than 6 months with no correlation between surgery timing and postoperative diplopia identified. With the prospective literature not sufficiently answering the question of timing, the investigators systematically examined retrospective studies comparing surgical timing. Fifteen studies were found that reported on surgical timing and various clinical outcomes. Of the 9 adult studies, 4 showed a significant positive effect on clinical outcomes (enophthalmos and ocular motility) with earlier surgery, whereas 5 others were inconclusive. In the pediatric orbital fracture studies, 1 showed a significant correlation between surgery within 3 weeks and diplopia long-term, whereas 5 others were not conclusive.

The review showed that the available data were insufficient to provide guidelines for the timing of orbital repair. It concluded that the evidence for early posttraumatic repair was limited to low-level evidence. The investigators called for quality prospective studies to help answer the important clinical question of the timing of repair.

In a companion systematic review, Dubois and colleagues[36] tried to identify which fracture size and fracture location should be repaired. This review looked at 231 studies that included more than 15,000 subjects. It found that 94% of the publications were retrospective studies describing a single institution's experience or were noncontrolled descriptions of a single treatment. The outcome measures were generally varied and subjective. Description of orbital fracture size and location were not clearly specified and many articles did not discuss complications. The review was able to identify only 14 prospective trials totaling 380 orbital fractures. Among these 14 studies, just 5 were controlled clinical trials, 4 of which were randomized. There was significant heterogeneity in the types and sizes of orbital fractures reported with only 1 randomized study describing both defect size and fracture location. Because of the small sample size of the studies and the poor descriptions of the fractures, the review could not draw any evidence-based conclusions for a defect-driven reconstruction. The question of what size and location of fractures require treatment remains unanswered in the literature.

There are also varying opinions as to what material is best for orbital repair. Generally, the fracture size (area of the defect or the orbital volume change) is the key element in choosing an orbital implant. Although small defects can heal with scar, larger defects probably require more rigid support to maintain or restore orbital volume and avoid enophthalmos. However, there are few suggestions in the literature concerning orbital repair materials and clinical outcomes to help guide the surgeon treating these injuries. There has also been recent interest in incorporating preoperative planning and intraoperative imaging and navigation into the management of orbital fracture repair. There are no prospective studies to determine if the benefits of these technologies warrant the increased cost. Until better evidence is available from the literature, surgeons will continue to rely on clinical experience and the available lower level studies to determine treatment.

Midface Fractures

Injuries of the central third of the face are relatively common and include Le Fort type maxillary fractures and zygomatico-maxillary complex fractures (ZMC). The management of these fractures has evolved greatly during the past 3 decades because lower profile miniplates allowing stable fixation of precisely reduced fractures became available. There is virtually no higher level literature to guide the surgeon in treatment of these Le Fort fractures. There are only retrospective case series and technique papers that focus on these fractures. The plating requirements for these injuries are still dictated by the experience of the treating surgeon.

The goal of treatment of a ZMC fracture is to restore the bone to its preinjury location and maintain orbital volume, thereby enhancing both the functional and cosmetic outcome.[37] There is debate about how much hardware is needed to accomplish this goal. Surgeons have observed that 3-point fixation of the ZMC (frontal-zygomatic suture, inferior orbital rim, and zygomaticomaxillary buttress) provides the greatest stability. However, some surgeons contend that fixation with 2 plates (fronto-zygomatic suture and zygomaticomaxillary buttress), and even 1 plate, can be sufficient if properly applied. A limited surgery with less hardware can result in shorter operative times, lower costs, and fewer complications. Like nearly all other aspects of facial trauma, there is limited evidence to direct the surgeon in this matter. In the only randomized study of zygoma fractures, Rana and colleagues[38] compared 2-point internal fixation to 3-point internal fixation. In this study of 100 subjects undergoing zygoma fracture repair, better malar projection and less vertical dystopia was seen after 3-point fixation. They also determined that the 3-point constructs were much more likely to be deemed stable. Based on these findings, the investigators recommended 3 points of fixation for all displaced ZMC fractures. Because this is the only study, additional work is needed to corroborate these results. Until then, clinical management will continue to be guided by surgeon experience.

Skull Base Fractures

Frontal sinus and naso-orbital ethmoid fractures are among the most challenging in facial trauma. Given a lower overall incidence, the management of these fractures has not been investigated by clinical trials. Instead, the literature consists almost entirely of case series and case studies in which management continues to be debated. There are many proposed algorithms to treat these complex injuries and avoid potentially catastrophic complications. There is no consensus for surgical indications, surgery timing, method of repair, or postoperative surveillance for frontal sinus fracture. The basic goal is creation of a safe sinus. Surgeons try to reestablish the frontal bony contour and maintain normal sinus function, which includes patent sinus outflow. When an injury makes assuring the patency of sinus outflow unlikely, it becomes necessary to eradicate the sinus and create a barrier between the intracranial and extracranial compartments. Recent advances and new surgical techniques have permitted traditional obliteration and cranialization techniques to be replaced by more conservative management.[39,40] These newer methods use endoscopic sinus surgery to preserve the frontal sinus and avoid complications. Given the low incidence of these injuries and an even lower rate of complications, an evidence-based approach to determine if or when obliteration or cranialization is appropriate would take decades.

Skull base fractures and other infrequent facial injuries point to some of the limitations inherent in relying on high-level evidence gained by randomized trials to answer important facial trauma questions. These relatively rare events may be better studied with other methods.

FUTURE DIRECTIONS

Although the RCT is the preferred experimental design, significant obstacles limit reliance on these studies to determine the best practices for facial trauma. Injuries that occur infrequently and injuries that have many concurrent variables make RCTs impractical or impossible. Several other areas of medicine have developed expanded clinical registries that allow auditing of clinical standards and quality assessments.[41,42] These registries combined with the electronic medical record can provide a large amount of observational data. These data are used to supplement the conclusions drawn and allow researchers to identify topic areas for which a focused RCT is needed. Finally, registries also help overcome some of the shortfalls of randomized trials by allowing accrual of clinical data at multiple sites prospectively. Because results from small RCTs are accentuated in meta-analysis, data from a heterogynous population help offset some of the problems encountered for conditions that are so infrequent that a trial is not possible. There has been interest in establishing registries for facial trauma. Several European trauma centers recently joined together and are prospectively compiling facial trauma demographic data.[43] This European Maxillofacial Trauma (EUMAT) project is attempting to combine resources to better identify future clinical and research priorities. Such efforts are certain to improve the quality of the facial trauma literature.

SUMMARY

There is limited higher level evidence available to surgeons treating facial trauma management. Although there have been improvements in the quality and level of evidence, it is still predominantly lower level. This does not mean that surgeons should minimize the contributions these retrospective series have made in the understanding of facial fracture management. Despite the methodological faults, these less rigorous studies are, at times, the only research available to answer a clinical question. With the goal of providing the best care to patients, surgeons have an obligation to attempt randomized trials to investigate important clinical questions. When such trials are impractical, using multiinstitutional clinical registries can enhance the understanding of treatment outcomes and help satisfy the goal of using an evidence-based approach to treatment.

REFERENCES

1. Andreasen JO, Jensen SS, Schwartz O, et al. A systematic review of prophylactic antibiotics in the surgical treatment of maxillofacial fractures. J Oral Maxillofac Surg 2006;64:1664–8.
2. Kyzas PA. Use of antibiotics in the treatment of mandible fractures: a systematic review. J Oral Maxillofac Surg 2011;69:1129–45.
3. Miles BA, Potter JK, Ellis E. The efficacy of postoperative antibiotic regimens in the open treatment of mandibular fractures: a prospective randomized trial. J Oral Maxillofac Surg 2006;64:576–82.
4. Shridharani SM, Berli J, Manson PN, et al. Evidence-based medicine versus experience-based medicine in plastic surgery: The role of postoperative antibiotics in mandible fractures - a systematic review of the literature and international survey. Ann Plast Surg 2014. [Epub ahead of print].
5. Knepil GJ, Lakouta RA. Outcomes of prophylactic antibiotics following surgery for zygomatic bone fracture. Journal of Cranio-maxillo-facial Surgery 2010;38:131–3.
6. Morris LM, Kellman RM. Are prophylactic antibiotics useful in the management of facial fractures? Laryngoscope 2014;124:1282–4.
7. Brodie HA. Prophylactic antibiotics for posttraumatic cerebrospinal fluid fistulae. A meta-analysis. Arch Otolaryngol Head Neck Surg 1997;123:749–52.
8. Villalobos T, Arango C, Kubilis P, et al. Antibiotic prophylaxis after basilar skull fractures: a meta-analysis. Clin Infect Dis 1998;27:364–9.
9. Ratilal BO, Costa J, Sampaio C, et al. Antibiotic prophylaxis for preventing meningitis in patients with basilar skull fractures. Cochrane Database Syst Rev 2011;(8):CD004884.
10. Mondin V, Rinaldo A, Ferlito A. Management of nasal bone fractures. Am J Otolaryngol 2005;26:181–5.
11. Fernandes SV. Nasal fractures: the taming of the shrewd. Laryngoscope 2004;114:587–92.
12. Staffel JG. Optimizing treatment of nasal fractures. Laryngoscope 2002;112:1709–19.
13. Khwaja S, Pahade AV, Luff D, et al. Nasal fracture reduction: local versus general anesthesia. Rhinology 2007;45:83–8.
14. Chadha NK, Repanos C, Carswell AJ. Local anaesthesia for manipulation of nasal fractures: systematic review. J Laryngol Otol 2009;123:830–6.
15. Atighechi S, Baradaranfar MH, Akbari SA. Reduction of nasal bone fractures: a comparative study of general, local, and topical anesthesia techniques. J Craniofac Surg 2009;20:382–4.
16. Al-Moraissi EA, Ellis E. Local versus general anesthesia for the management of nasal bone fractures: a systematic review and meta-analysis. J Oral Maxillofac Surg 2015;73(4):606–15.
17. Danda AK. Comparison of a single noncompression miniplate versus 2 noncompression miniplates in the treatment of mandibular angle fractures: a prospective, randomized clinical trial. J Oral Maxillofac Surg 2010;68:1565–7.
18. Siddiqui A, Markose G, Moos KF, et al. One miniplate versus two in the management of mandibular angle fractures: a prospective randomized study. Br J Oral Maxillofac Surg 2007;45:223–5.
19. Laverick S, Siddappa P, Wong H, et al. Intraoral external oblique ridge compared with transbuccal lateral cortical plate fixation for the treatment of fractures of the mandibular angle: prospective randomised trial. Br J Oral Maxillofac Surg 2012;50:344–9.
20. Sugar AW, Gibbons AJ, Patton DW, et al. A randomised controlled trial comparing fixation of mandibular angle fractures with a single miniplate placed either transbuccally and intra-orally, or intra-orally alone. Int J Oral Maxillofac Surg 2009;38:241–5.
21. Adeyemi MF, Adeyemo WL, Ogunlewe MO, et al. Is healing outcome of 2 weeks intermaxillary fixation different from that of 4 to 6 weeks intermaxillary fixation in the treatment of mandibular fractures? J Oral Maxillofac Surg 2012;70:1896–902.
22. Kaplan BA, Hoard MA, Park SS. Immediate mobilization following fixation of mandible fractures: a prospective, randomized study. Laryngoscope 2001;111:1520–4.
23. Nasser M, Pandis N, Fleming PS, et al. Interventions for the management of mandibular fractures. Cochrane Database Syst Rev 2013;(7):CD006087.
24. Dorri M, Nasser M, Oliver R. Resorbable versus titanium plates for facial fractures. Cochrane Database Syst Rev 2009;(1):CD007158.
25. Ahmed W, Gulzar S, Bukhari A, et al. Bioresorbable versus titanium plates for mandibular fractures. J Coll Physicians Surg Pak 2013;23:480–3.
26. Eckelt U, Schneider M, Erasmus F, et al. Open versus closed treatment of fractures of the mandibular condylar process—a prospective randomized

multi-centre study. J Craniomaxillofac Surg 2006;34: 306–14.

27. Singh V, Bhagol A, Goel M, et al. Outcomes of open versus closed treatment of mandibular subcondylar fractures: a prospective randomized study. J Oral Maxillofac Surg 2010;68:1304–9.

28. Danda AK, Muthusekhar MR, Narayanan V, et al. Open versus closed treatment of unilateral subcondylar and condylar neck fractures: a prospective, randomized clinical study. J Oral Maxillofac Surg 2010;68:1238–41.

29. Kotrashetti SM, Lingaraj JB, Khurana V. A comparative study of closed versus open reduction and internal fixation (using retromandibular approach) in the management of subcondylar fracture. Oral Surg Oral Med Oral Pathol Oral Radiol 2013;115:e7–11.

30. Nussbaum ML, Laskin DM, Best AM. Closed versus open reduction of mandibular condylar fractures in adults: a meta-analysis. J Oral Maxillofac Surg 2008;66:1087–92.

31. Sharif MO, Fedorowicz Z, Drews P, et al. Interventions for the treatment of fractures of the mandibular condyle [review]. Cochrane Database Syst Rev 2010;(4):CD006538.

32. Liu Y, Bai N, Song G, et al. Open versus closed treatment of unilateral moderately displaced mandibular condylar fractures: a meta-analysis of randomized controlled trials. Oral Surg Oral Med Oral Pathol Oral Radiol 2013;116:169–73.

33. Schmelzeisen R, Cienfuegos-Monroy R, Schön R, Chen CT, et al. Patient benefit from endoscopically assisted fixation of condylar neck fractures—a randomized controlled trial. J Oral Maxillofac Surg 2009;67:147–58.

34. Ridgway EB, Chen C, Colakoglu S, et al. The incidence of lower eyelid malposition after facial fracture repair: a retrospective study and meta-analysis comparing subtarsal, subciliary, and transconjunctival incisions. Plast Reconstr Surg 2009; 124:1578–86.

35. Dubois L, Steenen SA, Gooris PJJ, et al. Controversies in orbital reconstruction—II. Timing of post-traumatic orbital reconstruction: a systematic review. Int J Oral Maxillofac Surg 2015;44(4):433–40.

36. Dubois L, Steenen SA, Gooris PJJ, et al. Controversies in orbital reconstruction—I. Defect-driven orbital reconstruction: a systematic review. Int J Oral Maxillofac Surg 2015;44(3):308–15.

37. Ellstrom CL, Evans GR. Evidence-based medicine: zygoma fractures. Plast Reconstr Surg 2013;132: 1649–57.

38. Rana M, Warraich R, Tahir S, et al. Surgical treatment of zygomatic bone fracture using two points fixation versus three point fixation—a randomised prospective clinical trial. Trials 2012;13:36.

39. Guy WM, Brissett AE. Contemporary management of traumatic fractures of the frontal sinus. Otolaryngol Clin North Am 2013;46(5):733–48.

40. Pawar SS, Rhee JS. Frontal sinus and naso-orbital-ethmoid fractures. JAMA Facial Plast Surg 2014; 16:284–9.

41. Quality assurance in surgical oncology the EURECCA platform [editorial]. Eur J Surg Oncol 2014; 40:1387–90.

42. Granan LP, Bahr R, Steindal K, et al. Development of a national cruciate ligament surgery registry. The Norwegian National Knee Ligament Registry. Am J Sports Med 2008;36:308–15.

43. Boffano P, Roccia F, Zavattero E, et al. European Maxillofacial Trauma (EURMAT) project: a multi-centre and prospective study. J Craniomaxillofac Surg 2015;43:62–70.

Microvascular Reconstruction
Evidence-Based Procedures

Steven B. Cannady, MD[a], Eric Lamarre, MD[b],
Mark K. Wax, MD[c],*

KEYWORDS

- Free flap • Reconstruction • Functional outcome • Monitoring • Mandible

KEY POINTS

- The goal of evidence-based medicine is to evaluate outcomes to provide improved care to patients.
- In the field of microvascular reconstruction, the level of evidence is mediocre.
- Monitoring of free flaps has allowed for improved outcomes and lower revision rates.
- Reconstruction with bony flaps for the lateral mandibular defect has proven to be efficacious.
- A collaborative, multiinstitutional study should be able to improve the level of evidence that exists.

INTRODUCTION

Evidence-based medicine integrates research, clinical expertise, and patient values.[1] It attempts to evaluate scientific evidence and clinical care experiences to provide a rationale for decision making in the care of patients. This contrasts with the tradition of treating patients as was learned in residency or fellowship. It strives to bring a rationale to the decision-making process as opposed to the commonly quoted, "In my experience." Finding good literature to make evidence-based decisions when it comes to operative procedures is difficult. Randomized, controlled studies, considered the best modality to amass evidence, are almost impossible to perform when comparing 2 different operative procedures, or across modalities of treatment focused on low volume-disease, such as head and neck cancer.[2] For a variety of reasons, we are often left with comparing different procedures as they have evolved in a single institution or with comparing results between institutions. Still, it is possible to use this broad-based information if we recognize the selection biases and the limitations of the data.

In this article, we present 3 areas in the field of microvascular reconstruction where data exist that allows one to make an evidence-based decision on clinical care. The first is postoperative monitoring of free tissue transfer. Although it seems logical and empiric that monitoring is a good thing to do, little clear-cut evidence exists as to its efficacy. Second, the reconstruction of lateral mandibular defects can be performed in a number of ways. Few comparative studies have been performed, yet some evidence does exist. Finally, functional outcomes are reported to be improved with free tissue transfer. Analysis of the individual surgeon or institutional evidence reveals superiority of free tissue over regional or local transfer, yet functional outcome reporting is inconsistent with most reports using nonvalidated instruments or custom designed assessment tools. Thus, this review sought to define the state of

The authors have no conflict of interest or financial disclosures to disclose.
[a] Department of Otolaryngology-HNS, University of Pennsylvania, Houston Hall, 3417 Spruce Street, Philadelphia, PA 19104, USA; [b] Department of Otolaryngology-HNS, Cleveland Clinic Foundation, 9500 Euclid Avenue, Cleveland, OH 44195, USA; [c] Department of Otolaryngology-HNS, Oregon Health and Sciences University, 3181 Southwest Sam Jackson Park Road PV-01, Portland, OR 97239, USA
* Corresponding author.
E-mail address: waxm@ohsu.edu

Facial Plast Surg Clin N Am 23 (2015) 347–356
http://dx.doi.org/10.1016/j.fsc.2015.04.007
1064-7406/15/$ – see front matter © 2015 Elsevier Inc. All rights reserved.

reporting for functional outcomes in head and neck reconstruction studies suggesting they provide function information, and assess quality of life (QOL) data between 2002 and 2012.

MONITORING FREE TISSUE TRANSFER

The ability to transfer successfully tissue from 1 part of the body to another is related to patient factors and the technical ability of the microvascular reconstructive surgeon. Total failure of the flap is a rare and devastating complication that is usually secondary to vascular anastomotic failure. This results in thrombosis of the anastomosis and death of the tissue. The need to reexplore microvascular anastomosis is consistently reported at between 10% and 12%[3–6] (level 4 evidence). When flaps are explored in a timely manner, successful revascularization is reported it up to 70% to 80% of cases. This led to a belief that monitoring of the tissue in the postoperative period should be intensive. Routines have involved clinical monitoring the flap hourly by medical personnel. The advent of resident duty-hour restrictions and improved technology has changed the paradigm so that nursing personnel primarily monitors the flap with medical input on a less frequent basis.

Clinical Monitoring Involving Evaluation of the Flap by Physical Examination

Looking for color, turgor, and warmth has been the mainstay of physical examination for many decades (**Fig. 1**). Even with this modality, the incidence of flap revision and ultimately survival has not changed[3,5,7–9] (level 4 evidence). This led to the desire to find technological methodologies to supplement the clinical examination. By far the most

common method used is the placement of an intraoperative Doppler monitor[7,10,11] (level 4 evidence).

The Doppler can be placed in a sheath around the artery or it can be used as part of an implantable coupling device (**Fig. 2**). Schmulder and colleagues in 2011[10] compared 259 patients monitored with the implantable Doppler and compared them with 289 patients monitored using clinical measures only (Level 3 Evidence). The patients monitored with the implantable Doppler had an overall survival rate that was significantly higher than those monitored clinically. The reexploration rate was also higher in the flaps with implantable Dopplers. The surgical salvage rate improved from 40% to 95% and the success rate improve from 84% to 95%. False positives occurred in 3 of 36 patients. In 2 of these, the patient was explored and the Doppler wire was dislodged. There were no false negatives. Most authors suggest that, when the Doppler suggests compromise and the clinical examination suggests a viable flap, careful and intensive observation can be performed after trouble shooting the device.

Wax[7] evaluated 1142 patients who had a Doppler placed in the intraoperative setting. They determined that 10% of patients develop intraoperative vascular problems that were successfully revised. Compared with contemporary literature with a reexploration rate of 10% to 14%, their postoperative revision rate was 7%. The majority of revisions were after 12 hours, in contradiction to the literature in which the majority of revisions are within the first 12 hours. They felt that use of the Doppler in the intraoperative setting allowed them to detect issues with the vascular anastomosis that would have been undetected until the patient was in the recovery room or on the ward. They also demonstrated that the patients who had intraoperative vascular issues were more likely to suffer postoperative issues with a lower salvage rate.

Overall, this seems to indicate that monitoring of free flaps for vascular compromise in the intraoperative and postoperative setting is beneficial to patient care. The detection of vascular compromise allows for an active intervention with salvage in a significant number of patients (level 4 evidence).

LATERAL MANDIBULAR DEFECT

Reconstruction of the mandible continues to be a challenging problem faced by reconstructive surgeons. Techniques have evolved over the last century. The mandibular swing was the standard operation with adequate, although improvable, healing and functional outcomes. The cosmetic outcomes were poor and dental rehabilitation was not possible (**Fig. 3**). The introduction of rigid

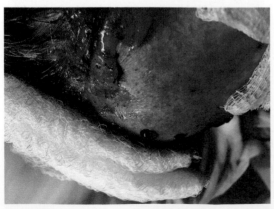

Fig. 1. Flap with signs of vascular compromise. It is blue, turgid, and was very swollen. Notice the dark blood at the needle prick site.

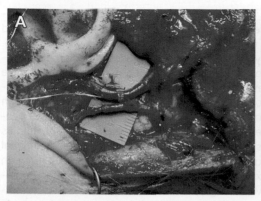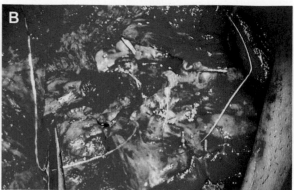

Fig. 2. A doppler probe is used. (*A*) Here it has been placed around the artery. (*B*) Here it has been incorporated into the flow coupler and monitors the vein.

fixation allowed surgeons to improve rehabilitation. With improved materials, a lateral mandibular defect could be reconstructed safely with local tissue transfer and a plate. Although this had proved to be successful in many cases, over time extrusion or fracture of the plate would happen[12] (level 4 evidence). The patients were also unable to undergo full dental rehabilitation and plate extrusion rates were higher than was desirable. Reconstruction continued to evolve and free tissue transfer allowed for the replacement of the composite bony defect, allowing for oral and dental rehabilitation. It is now purported that bony reconstruction is the "gold" standard[13] (level 3 evidence).

The choice of which osteocutaneous free tissue transfer to use has been complex. For lateral mandibular defects, the radial forearm osteocutaneous (**Fig. 4**), the fibula osteocutaneous (**Fig. 5**), and scapula osteocutaneous (**Fig. 6**) are most commonly used[14–16] (level 3 and level 4 evidence). The fibula osteocutaneous free flap his evolved as the best reconstructive modality owing to its ability to handle dental implants and thus improve dental

rehabilitation. Although this is stated empirically, it has been difficult to prove. The study by Dean and colleagues[17] (level 3 evidence) compared outcomes of patients reconstructed with radial forearm osteocutaneous flaps as opposed to the fibula osteocutaneous flap. They determined that the outcome was equivalent between both groups in terms of postoperative diet, return of oral function, and oral rehabilitation. Others have substantiated this result. Interestingly, none of the fibula patients obtained implants for dental rehabilitation and only a few obtained dentures. This demonstrated the disconnect seen between theoretic benefits as speculated on by the surgeon and what patients are willing to follow through on. Although mandibular reconstruction with free tissue transfer is the best option for healing, oral rehabilitation, and cosmesis in this patient population, the goal of dental rehabilitation remains elusive. Whether a fibula or radial osteocutaneous flap provides the best reconstruction is unknown at this time. If dental implants are to be used, then the fibula is the best option; however, the data are lacking.

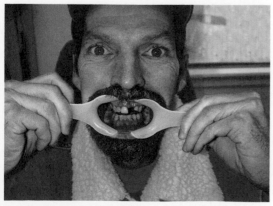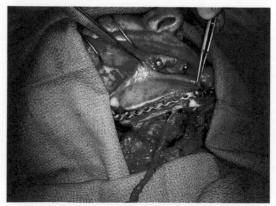

Fig. 3. This patient had a mandibulectomy with no mandible reconstruction. He was allowed to swing.

Fig. 4. A radial forearm osteocutaneous free flap has been used to reconstruct this lateral mandibular defect.

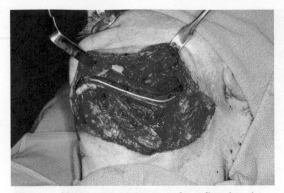

Fig. 5. A fibula osteocutaneous free flap has been used to reconstruct this lateral mandibular defect.

Functional Outcomes in Reconstruction of the Oral Cavity and the Oropharynx

The impact of microvascular free tissue transfer in reconstructing ablative defects of the oral cavity and the oropharynx has significantly shaped the surgical management of malignancies in these subsites.[18] With the proven reliability of free tissue transfer, the future emphasis will be on analyzing and optimizing function. Evaluations of functional outcomes are reported in several ways: (1) examination of a particular flap/technique in reconstructing defects, or (2) by evaluating a surgeon's experience with a flap or comparison of different flaps in reconstruction of similar defects. Within these studies, there is a diversity of metrics ranging from aesthetic-related questions and functional objective data to QOL questionnaires. Furthermore, the consistency of metrics is variable, ranging from self-created outcome measures to validated instruments. In general, there is a lack of clear consensus on which measures to use; as a result, comparisons between studies is challenging.

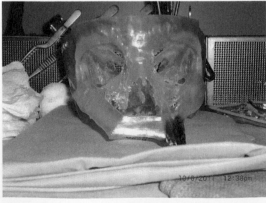

Fig. 6. A scapula osteocutaneous free flap has been used to reconstruct this lateral mandibular defect.

Systematic reviews are structured literature reviews characterized by robust methodology and a focused research question[19] (level 5 evidence). Systematic reviews in head and neck reconstruction have increased in recent years, but a definitive review of the functional outcomes in reconstruction is lacking[20] (level 3 evidence). Although nonoperative management of head and neck cancers have well-designed, single-institution studies as well as systematic review to assess functional outcomes[21,22] (level 3 evidence), such rigor in examining the role of reconstruction in the operative management of this disease has not been employed. We asked the following question to guide our systematic review: what are the functional outcomes of head and neck reconstruction involving the oral cavity and oropharynx? The primary aim of the review was to understand the functional implications involving reconstructions of the oral cavity and oropharynx; the secondary aim was to examine the metrics used in examining functional outcomes. Our objective was to assess the current state of research regarding functional outcomes in reconstruction of oral cavity and oropharyngeal defects, assess the limitations of the studies, and propose recommendations on how to guide further research on functional outcomes.

Historically, free tissue reconstruction after ablative surgery was thought to be associated with worse functional outcome than primary closure. McConnel and colleagues[23] argued that oropharyngeal defects were best closed with a primary closure. However, close inspection of the data reveals that the defect volume/reconstruction volume was higher in local reconstruction versus free tissue; this technique would leave a deficit even in resected and reconstructed beds that do not approximate functional needs as they are now understood. Free tissue should reconstitute at least the volume of lost tissue with some overcorrection to account for shrinking and radiation change[23] (level 3 evidence).

Comparisons between regional flap reconstructions, such as pectoralis major flaps and free tissue for oral and oropharynx sites, reveal superiority of free tissue[24] (level 3 evidence). Hsing and colleagues[24] compared QOL outcomes in 491 consecutive patients undergoing resection and regional transfer to free tissue reconstruction of the oral cavity. Applying the University of Wisconsin QOL survey, they were able to demonstrate that patients receiving free tissue rated their speech, mood, and shoulder function domains significantly better than those that had pectoralis rotation flaps. In addition Guerin-Lebailly and colleagues[25] showed that patient, family, and professional assessments of speech were superior in their cohort of free tissue reconstructed patients compared with local or regional tissues; sentence intelligibility, food score, and Hirose scoring outcome (a measure of speech function) were significantly better with free flaps for oral cavity defects (level 3 evidence). Markkanen-Leppanen and colleagues[26] in a series of studies further demonstrated that oral and oropharynx defects compromise velopalatal dynamics and alter speech articulations, but that free tissue can help to improve negative aspects. They also demonstrated that treatment negatively impacted QOL at 12 months, and this was reportedly associated with socioeconomic status. Specifically, voice quality remained the same after free tissue but articulations, particularly of /r/ and /s/ proved challenging.

Because free tissue has become the mainstay of oral and oropharynx upfront reconstructions, more literature has emerged reporting functional information. Complex interplay between tumor type, site, prior or future therapy, type of reconstruction, skill level of reconstructive surgeon, motivation of patient for rehabilitation, skill of speech therapist all affect the dynamic.

METHODOLOGY

We searched the electronic databases PubMed and Cochrane databases with MeSH terms: "oral cavity functional outcome free flap," "oropharynx functional outcome free flap," "oral cavity swallowing free flap," "oral cavity speech free flap," "oropharynx swallowing free flap," and "oropharynx speech free flap." Two reviewers (E.D.L. and S.B.C.) independently reviewed the abstracts and the selected papers. Furthermore, bibliographies from the searched articles were examined and additional titles were included if they were not a part of original search.

Inclusion Criteria

Studies included those written in English. Selected papers were written between January 1, 2002, and December 31, 2012, focusing on functional outcomes in patients undergoing reconstruction of oral cavity or oropharyngeal defects. The papers had the ablative defects and the types of free flap used clearly defined. Also, the outcomes studied were described clearly in the methodology. Retrospective, prospective, single-institution, and multiinstitution studies were included.

Exclusions

Series with fewer than 20 patients and papers with nondistinguishable outcome measures were excluded. Studies where the focus was not functional outcomes were also excluded from the review. Studies with duplicated patient cohorts were also excluded (ie, a second paper with increased numbers was used over predecessor paper).

Data extracted from individual studies included study type (based on Oxford CEBM levels of evidence), ages, male to female ratio, median follow-up time, adjuvant treatments, functional metrics used, and QOL surveys used.

RESULTS

In total, 358 papers were identified in our search. From this group, 112 abstracts were included and 246 abstracts were excluded. Of the 112 papers that were reviewed, an additional 44 papers were excluded and an additional 6 papers were added from the bibliography review, leaving a total of 74 papers reviewed (Fig. 7).

Data collected were broadly separated into swallowing outcomes, QOL metrics collected, and speech outcomes. The incidence of reporting on these outcomes is presented in Figs. 8–10. Studies that evaluated the University of Wisconsin QOL instrument are summarized in Table 1 with outcomes they analyzed.

DISCUSSION

When comparing different modalities of treatment, locoregional control and overall survival are critical parameters to assess equivalence. Because studies have cited the equivalence between surgery and nonsurgical treatments for oropharyngeal malignancies, reported functional outcomes and expectations can help patients to navigate complex treatment-related decisions[27] (level 3 evidence). Although the gains of microvascular surgery in the management of cancers of the oral cavity and oropharynx have been well-documented, the functional implications of reconstruction are not as well-defined. In addition, maturing functional data emerging from radiation oncology studies have set the precedent that these data will be used to help determine optimal therapies for given tumor locations[28] (level 4 evidence). Therefore, as the resurgence in surgical

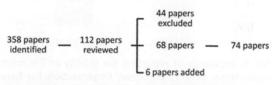

Fig. 7. Flow chart of papers identified and used.

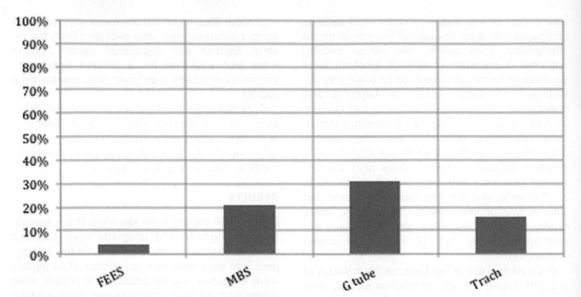

Fig. 8. Incidence of reporting for swallowing outcomes in papers reviewed. FEES, fiberoptic endoscopic evaluation of swallowing; G-tube, dependence on feeding tube; MBS, modified barium swallow; Trach, dependence on tracheostomy tube.

management of oropharynx tumors continues, it is incumbent upon the surgeon to demonstrate that function can parallel or improve upon nonsurgical data. Coincidently, recent interest in the nonsurgical management of oral cavity tumors requires the same rigorous functional assessment.

Overall, there is tremendous heterogeneity within studies reporting the functional outcomes of oral cavity and oropharyngeal free flaps as evidenced

by this review. This heterogeneity renders comparisons between the studies challenging. This heterogeneity exists along multiple facets: defect classification, adjuvant treatments, and the metrics used to measure functional outcomes.

The ability to accurately assess and compare functional outcomes between studies and across modality relies on accurate classification of defects (surgical or radiation leave field). The Brown

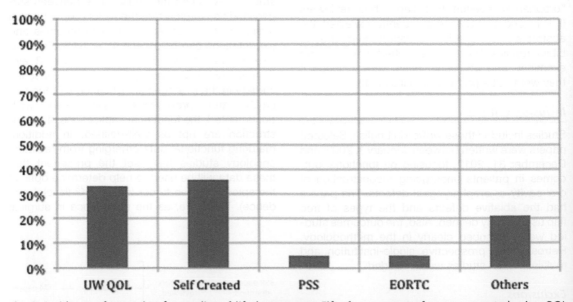

Fig. 9. Incidence of reporting for quality of life instruments. Fifty-four percent of papers reported using QOL evaluations. EORTC, European Organization for Research and Treatment of Cancer; PSS, performance status score; UW-QOL, University of Washington Quality of Life survey.

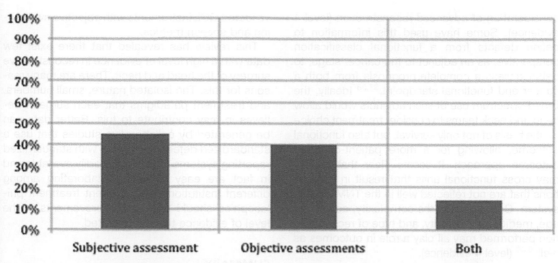

Fig. 10. Incidence of reporting of speech outcomes.

Classification of maxillectomy defects serves as a useful model in comprehensively classifying ablative defects and the challenges a reconstructive surgeon faces.[29] Defect classification systems exist for oral cavity and oropharyngeal defects, but are not used commonly.[30] Comparison between different techniques or types of flaps requires a common language to reference ablative defects.

Previous studies document that the outcomes in specific areas of the aerodigestive tract result in higher rates of aspiration, and speech and swallowing dysfunction that may not definitively overlap

with the TNM staging system[31,32] (level 4 evidence). For example, Khariwala and colleagues[31] showed that floor of mouth and central tongue base defects can be problematic functionally without being of an advanced stage. In addition, they showed that prior radiotherapy, total glossectomy, and hypopharynx site tumors lead to less likelihood of swallowing function. Furthermore, Genden and colleagues[33–36] have shown that defects that cross units of the oropharynx, such as base of tongue and soft palate, have an higher incidence of swallowing dysfunction and necessitate

Table 1
Sample of studies applying the UW-QOL survey to their functional outcomes studies with outcomes

Author, Year	Site	Domains with Effect	Outcome
Hsing et al,[24] 2011	OC	Physical function and social–emotional	Advanced T, radiotherapy, free flap needed worse QOL
Rogers, 2010	OCOP	Mood, shoulder, speech	Free flap better QOL
Kim, 2008	OP	Swallowing	Modification of RFFF improved score
Villaret, 2008	OC	Total score	Free flap better QOL vs pedicled flap
Thomas, 2009	OP	Speech	Free flap patients worse
Thomas, 2008	OP	Swallowing	Free flap patients swallow well, radiotherapy worsens
Markkanen-Leppanen et al,[26] 2006	OCOP	Total score	Complications affect recreation and chewing
Zuydam, 2005	OCOP	Speech and swallowing	Free flap needed worse outcome
Gabr, 2004	OC	Speech, swallowing, chewing	Percentage of patients 1–4 score
Rogers, 2004	OC	Overall	Bony flap worse scores than soft tissue Flap for segmental resection good outcomes

Abbreviations: OC, osteocutaneous; OCOP, oral cavity/oral pharynx; QOL, quality of life; RFFF, radial forearm free flap; T, tumor stage.

consideration of advanced reconstruction (level 4 evidence). Some have used this information to define defects from a functional classification perspective, as an adjunct to the cancer stage, to better assess a complete prognosis from both a cancer and functional standpoint.[37,38] Ideally, the broad-spectrum use of such adjuncts would allow head and neck teams to consider treatment choice on the basis of not only survival, but also functional outcome, allowing for a more patient-centered outcome approach. It seems clear that tumors may cross functional units that result in implications that are not reflected well in the TNM staging system. Compounding the complexity, advancing age, medical comorbidity, and type of reconstruction performed may all play a role in outcomes as well[39,40] (level 4 evidence).

Adjuvant treatment reporting is also critical in outcomes analyses. Surgery with radiation and chemotherapy invariably affect patient function and QOL more than surgery or radiation alone[21,22,28,41] (level 4 evidence). Although pure comparison between modalities may not be feasible, acknowledging the effects of adjuvant treatments have on function and QOL is important. For instance, a base of tongue defect reconstructed with a free flap will presumably have different functional results in comparison with a patient who undergoes the same reconstruction in a salvage setting. In addition, a patient treated with single modality trans oral robotic surgery (TORS) surgery may differ in function from one that requires postoperative radiation with or without chemotherapy.[42]

Depending on location, emphasis on function is characterized by specific subsite features with QOL relevant to all. Each site within the oral cavity and oropharynx has different goals of reconstruction with overlapping aspects that include both aesthetics and function. For example, patients with anterior mandibular and floor of the mouth tumors have challenges to their swallowing coordination, but also their appearance, whereas a patient with a palate reconstruction is most concerned with swallowing and speech. Future emphasis on patient-centered outcomes will afford the reconstructive surgeon the ability to give better information to patients on their predicted function and appearance. Ideally, a subsite "map" that accounts for all these factors will emerge, allowing one to inform the patient what their chance of swallowing, speaking, and being satisfied with aesthetics will be with surgery and reconstruction versus radiation. Standard reporting for studies aiming to provide functional outcome data should optimally include stage, defect site, adjuvant treatment specifics, and validated QOL instruments with objective swallowing and speech metrics.

This review has revealed that there exist few data with a high level of evidence in reconstructive surgery of the head and neck. There are many reasons for this. The isolated nature, small numbers, and treatment paradigms that each surgeon believes in may contribute to this. Better data can be generated by collaborative studies that use a standardized defect description with standardized reporting systems. These are readily available and in fact are easy to use. Collaborating among different institutions with different treatment philosophies should allow for improvements in the level of evidence that is generated.

SUMMARY

The goal of evidence-based medicine is to evaluate outcomes to provide improved care to patients. In the field of microvascular reconstruction, this has been demonstrated in many ways. Monitoring of free flaps has allowed for improved outcomes and lower revision rates. Reconstruction with bony flaps for the lateral mandibular defect has proven to be efficacious. Whether 1 flap is superior to another is not known. A collaborative, multi institutional study should be able to improve the level of evidence that exists.

REFERENCES

1. Sackett DL, Rosenberg WM, Gray JA, et al. Evidence based medicine: what it is and what it isn't. Clin Orthop Relat Res 2007;455:3–5.
2. Concato J, Shah N, Horwitz RI. Randomized, controlled trials, observational studies, and the hierarchy of research designs. N Engl J Med 2000; 342(25):1887–92.
3. Suh JD, Sercarz JA, Abemayor E, et al. Analysis of outcome and complications in 400 cases of microvascular head and neck reconstruction. Arch Otolaryngol Head Neck Surg 2004;130(8):962–6.
4. Wax MK, Rosenthal E. Etiology of late free flap failures occurring after hospital discharge. Laryngoscope 2007;117(11):1961–3.
5. Smit JM, Acosta R, Zeebregts CJ, et al. Early reintervention of compromised free flaps improves success rate. Microsurgery 2007;27(7):612–6.
6. Hidalgo DA, Jones CS. The role of emergent exploration in free-tissue transfer: a review of 150 consecutive cases. Plast Reconstr Surg 1990;86(3):492–8 [discussion: 499–501].
7. Wax MK. The role of the implantable Doppler probe in free flap surgery. Laryngoscope 2014;124(Suppl 1):S1–12.

8. Disa JJ, Cordeiro PG, Hidalgo DA. Efficacy of conventional monitoring techniques in free tissue transfer: an 11-year experience in 750 consecutive cases. Plast Reconstr Surg 1999;104(1):97–101.

9. Brown JS, Devine JC, Magennis P, et al. Factors that influence the outcome of salvage in free tissue transfer. Br J Oral Maxillofac Surg 2003;41(1):16–20.

10. Schmulder A, Gur E, Zaretski A. Eight-year experience of the Cook-Swartz Doppler in free-flap operations: microsurgical and reexploration results with regard to a wide spectrum of surgeries. Microsurgery 2011;31(1):1–6.

11. Kind GM, Buntic RF, Buncke GM, et al. The effect of an implantable Doppler probe on the salvage of microvascular tissue transplants. Plast Reconstr Surg 1998;101(5):1268–75.

12. Blackwell KE, Lacombe V. The bridging lateral mandibular reconstruction plate revisited. Arch Otolaryngol Head Neck Surg 1999;125(9):988–93.

13. Ch'ng S, Skoracki RJ, Selber JC, et al. Osseointegrated implant based dental rehabilitation in head and neck reconstruction patients. Head Neck 2014. [Epub ahead of print].

14. Virgin FW, Iseli TA, Iseli CE, et al. Functional outcomes of fibula and osteocutaneous forearm free flap reconstruction for segmental mandibular defects. Laryngoscope 2010;120(4):663–7.

15. Arganbright JM, Tsue TT, Girod DA, et al. Outcomes of the osteocutaneous radial forearm free flap for mandibular reconstruction. JAMA Otolaryngol Head Neck Surg 2013;139(2):168–72.

16. Militsakh ON, Werle A, Mohyuddin N, et al. Comparison of radial forearm with fibula and scapula osteocutaneous free flaps for oromandibular reconstruction. Arch Otolaryngol Head Neck Surg 2005; 131(7):571–5.

17. Dean NR, Wax MK, Virgin FW, et al. Free flap reconstruction of lateral mandibular defects: indications and outcomes. Otolaryngol Head Neck Surg 2012; 146(4):547–52.

18. Hanasono MM, Friel MT, Klem C, et al. Impact of reconstructive microsurgery in patients with advanced oral cavity cancers. Head Neck 2009; 31:1289–96.

19. Neely JG, Magit AE, Rich JT, et al. A practical guide to understanding systematic reviews and meta-analyses. Otolaryngol Head Neck Surg 2010;142:6–14.

20. Kreeft AM, van der Molen L, Hilgers FJ, et al. Speech and swallowing after surgical treatment of advanced oral and oropharyngeal carcinoma: a systematic review of the literature. Eur Arch Otorhinolaryngol 2009;266:1687–98.

21. Hunter KU, Lee OE, Lyden TH, et al. Aspiration pneumonia after chemo-intensity-modulated radiation therapy of oropharyngeal carcinoma and its clinical and dysphagia-related predictors. Head Neck 2014;36:120–5.

22. Hunter KU, Schipper M, Feng FY, et al. Toxicities affecting quality of life after chemo-IMRT of oropharyngeal cancer: prospective study of patient-reported, observer-rated, and objective outcomes. Int J Radiat Oncol Biol Phys 2013;85:935–40.

23. McConnel FM, Pauloski BR, Logemann JA, et al. Functional results of primary closure vs flaps in oropharyngeal reconstruction: a prospective study of speech and swallowing. Arch Otolaryngol Head Neck Surg 1998;124:625–30.

24. Hsing CY, Wong YK, Wang CP, et al. Comparison between free flap and pectoralis major pedicled flap for reconstruction in oral cavity cancer patients–a quality of life analysis. Oral Oncol 2011;47:522–7.

25. Guerin-Lebailly C, Mallet Y, Lambour V, et al. Functional and sensitive outcomes after tongue reconstruction: about a series of 30 patients. Oral Oncol 2012;48:272–7.

26. Markkanen-Leppanen M, Makitie AA, Haapanen ML, et al. Quality of life after free-flap reconstruction in patients with oral and pharyngeal cancer. Head Neck 2006;28:210–6.

27. de Almeida JR, Byrd JK, Wu R, et al. A systematic review of transoral robotic surgery and radiotherapy for early oropharynx cancer: a systematic review. Laryngoscope 2014;124:2096–102.

28. Eisbruch A, Kim HM, Feng FY, et al. Chemo-IMRT of oropharyngeal cancer aiming to reduce dysphagia: swallowing organs late complication probabilities and dosimetric correlates. Int J Radiat Oncol Biol Phys 2011;81:e93–9.

29. Brown JS, Rogers SN, McNally DN, et al. A modified classification for the maxillectomy defect. Head Neck 2000;22:17–26.

30. Urken ML, Weinberg H, Vickery C, et al. Oromandibular reconstruction using microvascular composite free flaps. Report of 71 cases and a new classification scheme for bony, soft-tissue, and neurologic defects. Arch Otolaryngol Head Neck Surg 1991; 117:733–44.

31. Khariwala SS, Vivek PP, Lorenz RR, et al. Swallowing outcomes after microvascular head and neck reconstruction: a prospective review of 191 cases. Laryngoscope 2007;117:1359–63.

32. Smith JE, Suh JD, Erman A, et al. Risk factors predicting aspiration after free flap reconstruction of oral cavity and oropharyngeal defects. Arch Otolaryngol Head Neck Surg 2008;134:1205–8.

33. de Almeida JR, Genden EM. Robotic assisted reconstruction of the oropharynx. Curr Opin Otolaryngol Head Neck Surg 2012;20:237–45.

34. de Almeida JR, Park RC, Genden EM. Reconstruction of transoral robotic surgery defects: principles and techniques. J Reconstr Microsurg 2012;28:465–72.

35. Genden EM, Kotz T, Tong CC, et al. Transoral robotic resection and reconstruction for head and neck cancer. Laryngoscope 2011;121:1668–74.

36. Genden EM, Park R, Smith C, et al. The role of reconstruction for transoral robotic pharyngectomy and concomitant neck dissection. Arch Otolaryngol Head Neck Surg 2011;137:151–6.

37. Nicoletti G, Soutar DS, Jackson MS, et al. Chewing and swallowing after surgical treatment for oral cancer: functional evaluation in 196 selected cases. Plast Reconstr Surg 2004;114:329–38.

38. Nicoletti G, Soutar DS, Jackson MS, et al. Objective assessment of speech after surgical treatment for oral cancer: experience from 196 selected cases. Plast Reconstr Surg 2004;113:114–25.

39. Dwivedi RC, St Rose S, Roe JW, et al. Validation of the Sydney Swallow Questionnaire (SSQ) in a cohort of head and neck cancer patients. Oral Oncol 2010; 46:e10–4.

40. Szczesniak MM, Maclean J, Zhang T, et al. The normative range for and age and gender effects on the Sydney Swallow Questionnaire (SSQ). Dysphagia 2014;29:535–8.

41. Ho KF, Farnell DJ, Routledge JA, et al. Comparison of patient-reported late treatment toxicity (LENT-SOMA) with quality of life (EORTC QLQ-C30 and QLQ-H&N35) assessment after head and neck radiotherapy. Radiother Oncol 2010;97: 270–5.

42. Weinstein GS, Quon H, O'Malley BW Jr, et al. Selective neck dissection and deintensified postoperative radiation and chemotherapy for oropharyngeal cancer: a subset analysis of the university of Pennsylvania transoral robotic surgery trial. Laryngoscope 2010;120:1749–55.

Cleft Lip and Palate
An Evidence-Based Review

David Shaye, MD[a], C. Carrie Liu, MD[b], Travis T. Tollefson, MD, MPH[c],*

KEYWORDS

- Cleft lip • Cleft palate • Evidence-based medicine • Outcomes

KEY POINTS

- The repair of unilateral cleft lip is performed using a rotation-advancement, geometric, straight-line, or hybrid technique.
- For bilateral cleft lip repair, most surgeons use either the Millard or Mulliken technique, and their variations.
- Most cleft centers perform cleft lip repair at the age of 3 to 5 months.
- Presurgical infant orthopedics, which can include nasoalveolar molding, is used before definitive cleft lip repair.
- For cleft palate repair, the 2-flap palatoplasty and Furlow double-opposing Z-plasty are most commonly used.

INTRODUCTION

At an estimated prevalence of 16.86 cases per 10,000 live births, isolated cleft palate, as well as cleft lip with or without cleft palate, is the most common congenital orofacial malformation in the United States.[1] Children with cleft anomalies may experience a multitude of physical and developmental challenges. There also may be psychosocial and emotional concerns for the patients and their families. As such, comprehensive care for the patient with cleft lip and/or palate requires an interdisciplinary team. The guidelines for team care outlined by the American Cleft Palate Association recommend team members that may include anesthesiology, audiology, genetics, neurosurgery, nursing, ophthalmology, oral maxillofacial surgery, orthodontics, otolaryngology–head and neck surgery, pediatrics, pediatric dentistry, physical anthropology, plastic surgery, prosthodontics, psychiatry, psychology, social work, and speech-language pathology.[2] Although every specialty may not be represented, the quality of care is augmented through collaborative discussion and coordination of care.

Broadly speaking, orofacial cleft anomalies may be unilateral or bilateral and involve the lip, the palate, or both. Although there have been considerable publications on this topic, most are single-surgeon/center experience papers or are retrospective in nature. As a result, the cleft lip–cleft palate literature regarding the clinical and surgical decision points lacks consensus. This review article seeks to define the typical management plans, describe the various viewpoints, and suggest recommendations based on the levels of evidence (**Table 1**) on the management of cleft lip

Funding sources: none.
Conflicts of interest: none.

[a] Division of Facial Plastic and Reconstructive Surgery, Massachusetts Eye & Ear Infirmary, Harvard Medical School, 243 Charles Street, Boston, MA 02114, USA; [b] Division of Otolaryngology – Head and Neck Surgery, Department of Surgery, Foothills Medical Centre, University of Calgary, 1403 - 29 Street Northwest, South Tower Room 602, Calgary, Alberta T2N 2T9, Canada; [c] Facial Plastic and Reconstructive Surgery, Department of Otolaryngology – Head and Neck Surgery, University of California, Davis, 2521 Stockton Boulevard, Suite 7200, Sacramento, CA 95817, USA
* Corresponding author.
E-mail address: travis.tollefson@ucdmc.ucdavis.edu

Facial Plast Surg Clin N Am 23 (2015) 357–372
http://dx.doi.org/10.1016/j.fsc.2015.04.008
1064-7406/15/$ – see front matter © 2015 Elsevier Inc. All rights reserved.

Table 1
Levels of evidence

Level I	High-quality, properly powered and conducted randomized controlled trial, systematic review, or meta-analysis of these studies
Level II	Well-designed controlled trial without randomization; prospective comparative cohort trial
Level III	Retrospective cohort study, case-control study, or systematic review of these studies
Level IV	Case series with or without intervention; cross-sectional study
Level V	Expert opinion, case reports, or bench research

Adapted from Oxford Centre for Evidence-Based Medicine. Available at: http://www.cebm.net/index.aspx?o51001. Accessed April 16, 2015.

and palate. The article is organized to address management of the techniques, timing, outcomes, and complications starting with cleft lip, and then addressing the same in cleft palate management.

CLEFT LIP
Overview

A typical orofacial cleft can be classified by *laterality*, *extent*, and *severity*. The *laterality* (left, right, asymmetric/symmetric bilateral) is noted with the unilateral deformity being more common than the bilateral. The *extent* of the cleft lip is variable and can include the cleft alveolus, which can be

complete or notched. Independent of the cleft lip type, the cleft palate is described as unilateral (one palatal shelf is attached to the nasal septum) or bilateral. The extent of the cleft is classified as complete (**Fig. 1**), incomplete (**Fig. 2**), or microform (**Fig. 3**). In the complete cleft, there is disruption of the lip's mucosal up to the nasal floor with the associated nasal deformity. There is a spectrum of incomplete clefting, ranging from vermilion notching to near-complete disruption of the lip with a remaining Simonart band.[3] An incomplete bilateral cleft lip can be quite asymmetric (**Fig. 4**). The *severity* of the cleft lip width can make the repair more difficult because of wound tension. Management of the more severe cleft lip often requires a more prolonged presurgical preparation period (eg, presurgical infant orthopedics [PSIO]).

In the complete unilateral cleft lip, there is an external and upward rotation of the medial segment of the premaxilla and an internal and posterior rotation of the lateral segment.[2] Fibers of the orbicularis oris muscle attach medially to the base of the columella and laterally to the alar base. The nasal septum is dislocated from the vomerian groove with a shortening of the columella. The alar cartilage of the cleft side is deformed such that the medial crus is displaced posteriorly and the lateral crus is flattened over the cleft.[2]

In the complete bilateral cleft lip deformity, the premaxilla and prolabium are entirely separate from the lateral lip and maxillary segments. As a result, the premaxilla protrudes past the lateral segments. The prolabium can vary in size and lacks the normal philtral structure of a central groove and philtral ridges. The vermilion cutaneous junction and cutaneous (white) roll are often

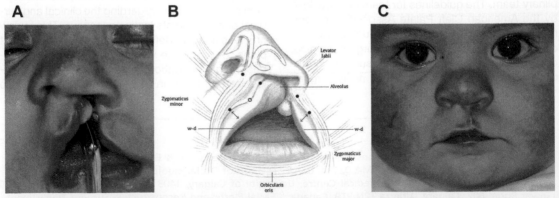

Fig. 1. Infant with unilateral complete cleft lip and palate. (*A*) Preoperative. (*B*) Illustration depicting the alveolus of the premaxilla, perioral muscles, and typical cleft nasal deformity. The arrows show the vermilion height, which should be made symmetric and the red line of Noordhoff (wet-dry junction) of the lip. (*C*) Postoperative view of same child after modified Mohler rotation-advancement repair and primary rhinoplasty. w-d, wet-dry vermillion. (*From* [*A*, *B*] Tollefson TT, Sykes JM. Unilateral cleft lip. In: Goudy S, Tollefson TT, editors. Complete cleft care. New York: Thieme; 2015. p. 40; with permission.)

A   **B**

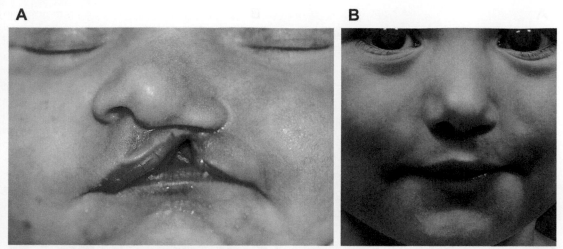

Fig. 2. Infant with incomplete cleft lip. (*A*) Preoperative. (*B*) Postoperative after a Fisher Subunit repair was used.

deficient. In a completed bilateral cleft lip, the prolabium does not contain orbicularis oris muscle. The nasal deformity associated with bilateral cleft lip is a shortened columella, flattened nasal tip, and alar hooding. Flaring of the alar base is common with inadequate alar base repair.[2]

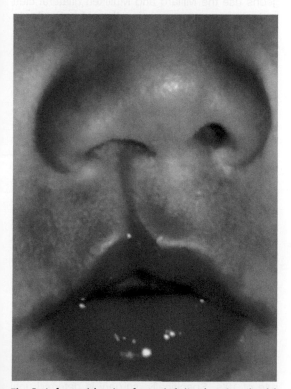

Fig. 3. Infant with microform cleft lip showing the (1) elevated Cupid peak, (2) furrowing of the philtrum, (3) medial dry vermilion deficient, (4) alar base malposition, (5) notched mucosa, and (6) deficient orbicularis oris muscle.

Surgical Techniques

Unilateral cleft lip

The objective of cleft lip repair is to approximate the medial and lateral lip elements with preservation of natural landmarks, align a functional concentric orbicularis, and to establish symmetry and proportionality. Unilateral cleft lip repair designs can be divided into 3 schools, which include (1) straight-line closure, (2) geometric, and (3) rotation-advancement techniques. The most common technique used to repair a unilateral cleft lip is the Millard rotation-advancement flap, as well as its modifications, including the Noordhoff vermilion flap and the Mohler modification.[3] There are few studies that compare the outcomes of various cleft lip repair techniques. Holtmann and Wray[4] (1983) studied patients randomized to receiving either the Millard rotation-advancement repair or the triangular (geometric) cleft lip repair, as described by Randall and colleagues[5] (Level II evidence). They did not find any significant differences in esthetic outcomes between the 2 groups. Chowdri and colleagues[6] (1990) also compared the Millard and Randall techniques in a randomized study (Level I evidence). Similar to Holtmann and Wray,[4] no differences were found in outcomes and both techniques were recommended in the repair of cleft lip.

There has been debate regarding whether the extent that the orbicularis oris muscles should be extensively released from the aberrant insertions on the maxilla to facilitate cleft lip repair. Some have felt that excessive dissection and a tense approximation of the muscular elements will lead to maxillary growth disturbance.[7] However, there is no evidence at present that muscular reconstruction leads to growth disturbance[8] (Level IV

A

B

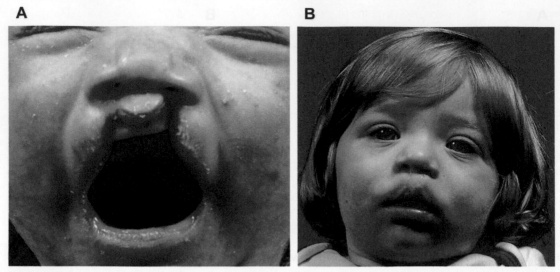

Fig. 4. (*A*) Two-week-old infant with asymmetric bilateral cleft lip and palate (incomplete on right and complete on left). (*B*) Six months postoperative.

evidence). In addition, the prevailing theory is that reconstructed musculature encourages normal and symmetric facial skeletal growth.[9,10] Two studies have suggested that muscular reconstruction leads to improved facial development[10,11] (Level II evidence). Although additional evidence is needed to conclude definitively regarding muscular reconstruction, it does seem to be associated with improved functional and esthetic outcomes.

Bilateral cleft lip

There are a few approaches to the repair of bilateral cleft lip. One approach is a 2-stage repair with columellar elongation as the second procedure between the ages of 1 and 5 years[12] (Level V evidence). Alternatively, a 1-stage approach with primary rhinoplasty at the time of cleft lip repair has been advocated for symmetric cases[13–15] (Level IV–V evidence).

The severely wide bilateral cleft lip with significantly projected premaxilla may necessitate with a staged cleft lip repair, PSIO, delayed repair, or premaxillary setback. In grossly asymmetric clefts or when a prolabium is less than 6 mm in height, a lip adhesion is performed, followed by a delayed definitive cleft lip repair, after the adhesion has successfully brought the soft tissue elements and maxillary arches closer together[16] (Level V evidence). Presurgical infant orthopedics, which includes nasoalveolar molding, is effective at decreasing the severity of the cleft width by applying orthopedic forces to the maxillary arches and premaxilla with an oral appliance.[17] Where presurgical infant orthopedics is ineffective or unavailable, premaxillary setback with vomer

osteotomy can be performed with caution. The risks of devascularizing the premaxilla as well as maxillary growth inhibition should be considered[18] (Level IV evidence). Most North American surgeons use the Millard and Mulliken bilateral cleft lip techniques or a variation thereof.[17] Similar to unilateral cleft lip repair, there is insufficient evidence to suggest the superiority of one technique over another.

Timing

There are advocates for cleft lip repair over a range of time frames, from the neonatal period to 5 to 6 months of age[19,20] (Level V evidence). Intrauterine repair has been piloted using animal models based on the potential benefit of no scar formation[21,22] (Level V evidence); however, this has not been seriously pursued in humans, as the theoretic benefits do not outweigh the risks of exposing both the mother and fetus to this procedure. Neonatal repair also has been investigated for the similar reasons of minimizing scar formation and potentially allowing molding of the nasal cartilages due to the intrauterine exposure to maternal hormones.[13] Earlier repair also has the proposed benefits of facilitating maternal-child bonding; however, studies have not been able to substantiate this[23] (Level V evidence).

In the absence of an obvious benefit with earlier repair, most surgeons adhere to the conventional rule of 10's. Specifically, surgery is deferred until the child is 10 pounds in weight, at or after 10 weeks of age, with a hemoglobin concentration of 10 g/dL.[24] This increases the safety of undergoing anesthesia. It also has been argued to improve esthetic results, as waiting allows for the lip musculature to grow[20,25] (Levels IV and V evidence).

Other Therapeutic Options

Presurgical infant orthopedics and nasoalveolar molding

Evidence supporting the use of PSIO is conflicting. This can likely be attributed to sparse evidence to definitively suggest a presurgical method is superior to another. Existing studies fail to use consistent outcome measures, which have partially driven the development of Eurocleft and Americleft research groups.[26] Two systematic reviews that examine the utility of PSIOs concluded that there is insufficient evidence to suggest an improvement in maxillary arch form/facial growth/occlusion, motherhood satisfaction, infant feeding/nutritional status, or speech[27,28] (Level II evidence).

Nasoalveolar molding (NAM) is a type of PSIO that incorporates the intraoral appliance with nostril prongs to improve the cleft nasal deformity (**Fig. 5**). There is more supportive evidence for PSIO due to the beginning of intraoral devices decades before NAM. Studies have shown that when instituted at 1 week of age and continued for 3 to 4 months, NAM is effective in approximating the cleft as well as improving the nasal deformity. Specifically, patients undergoing NAM treatment experienced improved nasal alar symmetry, columella lengthening, and nasal tip projection[29–32] (Levels II to V evidence). The counter arguments include nasal relapse and maxillary growth constriction. A recent

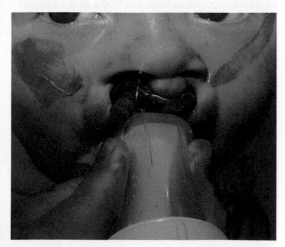

Fig. 5. Infant with left complete cleft lip and palate with NAM appliance. Tape will be secured into place with tape to the cheeks. Note the nasal prong that is expanded over time. This expands the soft tissue and cartilage, molding the nose before cleft lip repair. Also note the Haberman Feeder, allowing the parent to control the flow of formula into the mouth.

review concluded that there is some evidence for its use in the unilateral cleft population in improving nasal symmetry[33] (Level III evidence). Although randomized controlled trials at multi-institutional levels are lacking, there is evidence that NAM should be incorporated into the routine management of both unilateral and bilateral clefts. In a phone survey that contacted 89% of North American cleft centers, more than one-third of the centers offer NAM as an adjunct to surgical repair of unilateral and bilateral cleft lip.[3,34]

Lip adhesion

Lip adhesion surgery can be performed in unilateral and bilateral cleft lip. It is performed before definitive surgery, typically before 3 months of age. The rationale is that it applies orthopedic pressure on the underlying maxilla, thereby narrowing the cleft for the definitive repair[35,36] (Level V evidence); however, the evidence is limited and there is the potential disadvantage of additional scarring[37] (Level IV evidence).

Alveolar bone grafting

Primary alveolar bone grafting is typically performed at approximately 8 to 10 years of age. Some centers graft the alveolar cleft at age of 5 to 7 years, before the eruption of the permanent canines so as to improve bone height, dentofacial esthetics, and function[38] (Level IV evidence). Performing a primary graft in children younger than this is associated with the risk of insufficient alveolar bone volume. Bone grafting in older children may be associated with an increased risk of failure, as healing occurs more slowly and there is increased donor site morbidity[39] (Level II evidence). Iliac crest cancellous bone harvest is the standard, but other donor sites and off-label use of bone-morphogenetic protein have been described. More rarely described is the use of a split-rib technique with minimal maxillary dissection used for primary alveolar bone grafting, but the risks of maxillary growth restriction if performed too early must be considered[40] (Level IV evidence).

Primary rhinoplasty

A paradigm shift to include primary rhinoplasty at the time of cleft lip repair has been noted over the past few decades[41] (Level V evidence). Given the complexity of the nasal deformities associated with cleft lip, definitive rhinoplasty has and still is typically deferred until after adolescence and full skeletal growth[42] (Level V evidence). The rationale for minimal primary rhinoplasty during infancy was concern that significant change would occur during adolescent growth, necessitating repeat surgery.[43] There was also the theoretic risk of excessive scar tissue that would interfere with nasal growth. Finally, patients with cleft lip often require orthognathic surgery, which should precede definitive rhinoplasty.

Arguments against delaying rhinoplasty until adolescence are that waiting may lead to a worsened nasal deformity as well as symptoms of nasal obstruction and increased rates of revision surgery[44] (Level IV evidence). It also may be associated with psychological stress, given that patients will have to live with the unrepaired deformity until adolescence.[40] Over the past 3 decades, various investigators have published on their experiences with primary cleft rhinoplasty, demonstrating that stable long-term results can be achieved with minimal growth disturbance[45–53] (Level III–IV evidence). Therefore, some evidence does exist to support primary rhinoplasty in improving nasal appearance and function. A recent study showed that more than half of North American cleft surgeons do perform a limited rhinoplasty at the time of primary lip repair.[3]

Postoperative nasal stents

Nasal stents have been used for the goal of preventing secondary deformities with healing and scarring following primary repair (**Fig. 6**).[54] There have been case series, as well as one prospective study, demonstrating improved alar symmetry in those who underwent postoperative internal nostril stenting[54–56] (Level IV evidence). The limitations of using nasal stents include poor patient tolerance, possible airway distress in the case of stent dislodgement, and pressure ulcers.[55] Currently, there are no randomized controlled trials examining the benefits of postoperative nasal stenting.

Clinical Outcomes

There is significant variation among studies in measuring and reporting outcomes after cleft lip repair.[57] Some investigators have used clinical photographs with subjective scoring, whereas others use 3-dimensional imaging or anthropometry. The heterogeneity among patient populations, surgical techniques, and outcome assessment strategies make comparisons across studies difficult.

One outcome measure that can be used to gauge the success of cleft lip repairs is the rate of revision surgery. In a review of 50 consecutive patients with bilateral cleft lip with either a cleft palate or cleft alveolus, Mulliken and colleagues[58] found a nasolabial revision rate of 33% in the cleft lip and palate group (Level IV evidence). In the cleft lip and alveolus group, the revision rate was 12.5%. In a review of 750 patients with unilateral cleft lip, secondary reconstruction was performed in approximately 35% of patients[37] (Level IV evidence). The highest revision rates were reported by the Eurocleft study, which assessed the practice patterns and outcomes of 5 cleft centers in Northern Europe[59] (Level II evidence). Four centers provided revision rate data. One center reported a lip revision rate of 4%, and the remaining reported rates from 63% to 69%. For revision rates specific to nasal reconstruction, Mehrotra and Pradhan[60] reported a second rhinoplasty rate of 10% after primary rhinoplasty at the time of cleft lip repair (Level IV evidence).

Although revision rates provide a quantifiable method of gauging outcomes, it must be interpreted with caution. The decision to undertake revision surgery is family and surgeon-dependent. As such, the undertaking of revision surgery may be as reflective of these preferences as it is of the esthetic and functional outcomes from the primary repair. Furthermore, higher revision rates as an indicator of poorer outcome may not be accurate, as a child undergoing multiple revisions may actually have a final result that is more esthetically and functionally pleasing than a child who does not undergo any revisions.

Complications and Concerns

Wound complications

In a recent retrospective review of 3108 cases, Schonmeyr and colleagues[61] reported an overall short-term complication rate of 4.4% (Level IV

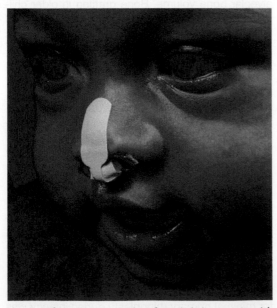

Fig. 6. Infant shown weeks after cleft lip repair with nasal conformers made of soft silicone secured in the nostrils. The optimal length of stenting the nostrils after primary rhinoplasty has not been established, but the senior author (TT) prefers 6 weeks.

evidence). In 0.5% of these cases, the complication was severe enough to warrant revision surgery. The most common early postoperative complications were wound dehiscence and/or infection, which were 4.3% in the previously mentioned study. This was consistent with the rates of 2.6% to 4.6% reported by other studies[26,62] (Level IV evidence). Complete clefts and bilateral clefts were both significantly associated with wound dehiscence[61] (Level IV evidence). Other complications included stitch granuloma (0.2%) and pressure necrosis (0.05%).

Maxillary growth

Concern also has been raised regarding cleft lip repair and effects on maxillary growth. There are various hypotheses for how lip repair can lead to maxillary retrusion. Some postulate that pressure from a repaired lip restricts maxillary growth[63,64] (Level V evidence). Maxillary growth restriction theoretically could be greater in complete cleft lip-palate as the maxillary segments would be less able to withstand the restrictive forces[65,66] (Level IV evidence). In a review of 82 patients with unilateral cleft lip, alveolus, and palate, lip repair was found to be associated with maxillary retrusion[67] (Level IV evidence). Those with more severe defects were found to have greater retrusion. In a prospective study of 22 patients with unilateral cleft lip and palate, lip repair was found to cause transverse narrowing of the maxilla without any effects on sagittal growth[68] (Level IV evidence).

CLEFT PALATE
Overview

A cleft deformity can occur in both the primary and secondary palates. Clefts of the primary palate range from an alveolar notch to those that extend through the hard and soft palates. Clefts of the secondary palate range from a bifid uvula to clefts that extend to the incisive foramen.[2] The soft palate consists of 5 muscles that are responsible for velopharyngeal closure, including the musculus uvulae, the palatoglossus, the palatopharyngeus, the tensor veli palatini, and the levator veli palatini. The levator veli palatini is the primary muscle involved in velopharyngeal closure. Normally, it originates from the Eustachian tube and inserts anteromedially onto the tensor aponeurosis, along with the tensor veli palatine.[69] In the cleft palate, the levator muscles insert aberrantly onto the posterior edge of the hard palate.[2] Contractions of the palatal muscles therefore become ineffective at closing the velopharynx.

Surgical Techniques

The goals of cleft palate repair include closure of the soft palate and reorientation of the levator veli palatini to obtain normal velopharyngeal closure and speech. Closure of the hard palate cleft separates the oral and nasal cavities. There are numerous techniques for cleft palate repair and there is significant variation in treatment protocols across cleft centers.[70]

One of the oldest procedures performed is the von Langenbeck palatoplasty. With this technique, bipedicled mucoperiosteal flaps are raised off of the hard palate. The cleft edges are incised and both nasal and oral mucosa are medialized. The biggest drawback to this technique is that it does not add additional length to the soft palate[20] (Level V evidence). Other techniques have been designed to improve velopharyngeal function by lengthening the velum. One such technique is the Veau-Wardill-Kilner palatoplasty, which is a variation of the V-Y pushback. Mucoperiosteal flaps are raised and retropositioned. This lengthens the velum but leaves a large area of exposed hard palate anteriorly, which heals by secondary intention. Variations of the V-Y pushback technique have fallen out of favor because of poor maxillary growth outcomes[20] (Level V evidence).

Two-flap palatoplasty (**Fig. 7**) was first introduced in 1967 by Bardach.[71] Large mucoperiosteal flaps based on the greater palatine vasculature are raised. Closure is layered to minimize tension, with approximation of the nasal and then oral mucosa. The soft palate musculature is then repaired via an intravelar veloplasty (IVV). IVV involves releasing the levator veli palatini from its aberrant attachment to the posterior hard palate. Among cleft surgeons, consensus is that IVV does improve velopharyngeal function and may reduce rates of secondary speech surgery; the drawbacks include additional operative time and devascularizing the muscle.[20] The muscle fibers are then reapproximated in the transverse direction to establish the palatal muscular sling.[20] Since its introduction, studies on the effectiveness of IVV have had conflicting but overall supportive results. Marsh and Galic[72] prospectively studied 51 patients randomized to receive or not receive IVV during cleft palate repair. In this study, IVV was not associated with improved speech (Level II evidence). On the contrary, a retrospective study of 213 patients showed that IVV improved speech and decreased the rate of secondary velopharyngeal insufficiency[73] (Level IV evidence). Neither study found an increased rate of complications with IVV. Other studies also have found improved

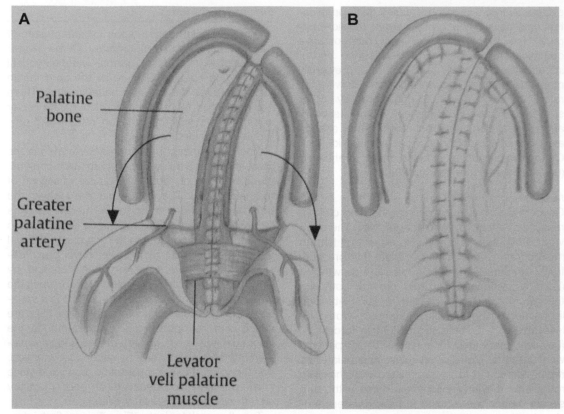

Fig. 7. Two-flap palatoplasty. (*A*) The flaps are elevated off the palatal bones and soft palate is dissected to create 2 flaps based off of the greater palatine neurovascular bundles. The orientation of the levator veli palatini muscles is corrected with or without a more extensive intravelar veloplasty. (*B*) A layered closure of the flap is then performed. (*From* Chiang T, Allen GC. Cleft palate repair. In: Goudy S, Tollefson TT, editors. Complete cleft care. New York: Thieme; 2015. p. 103; with permission.)

speech and velopharyngeal function with IVV[74,75] (Levels I and II evidence).

The Furlow double-opposing Z-plasty technique (**Fig. 8**) has gained popularity since its introduction in 1978. The soft palate is reapproximated in a way that lengthens it and realigns the musculature into a more anatomically correct position.[20] One concern raised with this technique is the increased rates of oronasal fistulas.[76] Only anecdotal evidence is available for the use of acellular dermis placed between the oral and nasal flaps to decrease in fistula rates[77,78] (Level IV evidence).

Studies have compared the various cleft repair techniques. Williams and colleagues[76] randomized patients to receive either a Furlow double-opposing Z-plasty or a von Langenbeck palatoplasty with IVV. Improved velopharyngeal function was found in the group that received the Furlow double-opposing Z-plasty (Level I evidence). Other studies also have found improved speech outcomes with the Furlow technique[79–81] (Level IV evidence). There is insufficient evidence to suggest a difference in outcomes between the Furlow technique and the 2-flap palatoplasty and a need for standardized speech outcomes collection to allow comparisons.

Timing
Evidence of the optimal timing of cleft palate repair remains inconclusive. Earlier repair provides the structural framework for speech development. Delaying repair may avoid potential maxillary growth inhibition. The consensus has leaned toward a timing of 10 and 14 months of age; however, evidence of alternative timing strategies deserve attention, including speech outcomes, maxillary growth, and staged soft palate/hard palate closure.

Speech Cleft palate surgery should occur early enough to facilitate optimal speech development. This means that repair should occur before the development of meaningful speech. Some have argued for palatoplasty no later than 13 months.[82] In a study by Dorf and Curtin,[83] 80 children underwent palate repair. Twenty-one of these children underwent repair earlier than 12 months of age

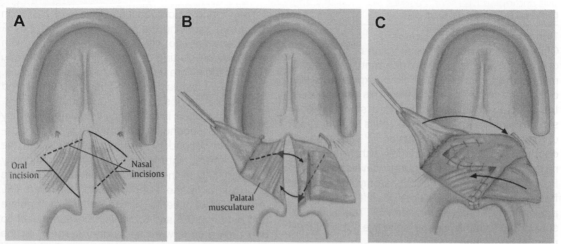

Fig. 8. Double-opposing Z-plasty (Furlow) palatoplasty. (*A*) Note that the left palate posteriorly based oral myo-mucosal layer is rotated posteriorly, whereas the left nasal mucosal layer is rotated anteriorly. (*B*) Conversely, the right anteriorly based mucosal layer is rotated anteriorly and the nasal myomucosal layer is rotated posteriorly. (*C*) This allows for the recreation of the levator sling and extends the palate posteriorly. (*From* Chiang T, Allen GC. Cleft palate repair. In: Goudy S, Tollefson TT, editors. Complete cleft care. New York: Thieme; 2015. p. 103; with permission.)

and the remainder underwent "late" repair, between 12 and 27 months. They found that children who underwent repair before 12 months of age exhibited better speech compared with those with late repair (Level IV evidence). In another study, by Pradel and colleagues,[84] 1-stage closure at 9 to 12 months of age was compared with 2-stage closure, with soft palate closure at 9 to 12 months of age and hard palate closure at 24 to 36 months. Again, 1-stage closure at 9 to 12 months was found to yield better speech development (Level IV evidence). Finally, Chapman and colleagues[85] found that children who underwent repair at the average age of 11 months had better speech outcomes compared with those who underwent repair at the average age of 15 months (Level IV evidence). The lack of consistent speech outcomes collection makes direct comparison between studies difficult.

Facial growth Cleft surgeons are concerned that dissection during palatoplasty disrupts the blood supply to the maxilla, leading to inhibited facial skeletal growth[86,87] (Level IV–V evidence). Studies investigating the effect of surgery on maxillary growth have had conflicting results, but often use dental arch models for comparisons and measurements. Chen and colleagues[88] compared sagittal maxillary growth in adults who had undergone palatal repair with those who had unrepaired cleft palates. They concluded that surgical trauma was not associated with more maxillary retrusion due to the similar retrusion between those with and without palatoplasty (Level IV evidence).

Alternatively, Ye and colleagues[89] found significant anterior dental arch constriction in those who had undergone a palatoplasty (Level IV evidence).

One-stage versus 2-stage (Schweckendiek) palate repair To mitigate the risk of growth interference, centers have experimented with 2-stage palate repairs with delayed hard palate closure.[90,91] An argument in favor of the 2-stage approach is that by performing a veloplasty first, the hard palate is encouraged to narrow. This allows for the use of smaller flaps at the time of the hard palate repair[92] (Level V evidence). Studies have supported the use of a 2-stage procedure as it facilitates normal midfacial growth[93–96] (Level IV evidence). However, delayed hard palate closure has been associated with a higher incidence of velopharyngeal insufficiency and compensatory misarticulations[97] (Level IV evidence).

With consideration of both speech and facial skeleton growth, most cleft centers perform 1-stage repair. As discussed previously, repair before the age of 15 months is associated with superior speech outcomes[83–85] (Level IV evidence). Kirschner and colleagues[98] investigated whether performing the repair before 7 months improved velopharyngeal function and speech and concluded that there is no benefit (Level IV evidence).

Summary Therefore, the current literature supports timing of the surgery to be between 7 to 15 months of age.[20] Steps taken to optimize maxillary growth include minimizing subperiosteal dissection and reducing exposure of the hard palate[99] (Level IV evidence).

Other Therapeutic Options

Tympanostomy tube placement

Cleft palate can affect the function of the Eustachian tube in part due to aberrant veli palatini muscular attachments and direct exposure of the oral cavity to the nasopharynx. This predisposes the affected child to middle ear dysfunction and subsequent recurrent acute otitis media and chronic otitis media with effusion.[100] The resultant conductive hearing loss carries with it concerns regarding speech and language development.[101] For these reasons, tympanostomy tubes are frequently placed at the time of cleft lip repair or palatoplasty[102] (Level III evidence). The evidence supporting routine versus selective tube placement is conflicting.

Aside from evaluating hearing status and presence or absence of middle ear pathology/effusions, the otolaryngologist must gather the evidence and provide direct clinical correlation. The routine use of tympanostomy tubes may prevent chronic ear effusions and the associated conductive hearing loss, but this is currently a matter of clinical controversy. Ponduri and colleagues[103] completed a systematic review of studies and divided these between *routine* (at palatoplasty) compared with *selective* placement of tympanostomy tubes in children with cleft palate. A paucity of quality randomized controlled trials were available, but routine placement in the neonatal period did not seem to be indicated. (Level II evidence). This is contradicted by the practice patterns of many cleft teams, who tend to place the first set of tympanostomy tubes at the time of the cleft lip repair.[37] Further studies are needed to address this complex clinical dilemma, as the children with cleft palate are an at-risk population regarding speech development. Providing the maximal hearing potential for these children while they develop speech may warrant more aggressive treatment than for children without clefts.

Clinical Outcomes

The outcomes of cleft palate repair can include fistula occurrence, speech outcomes (eg, resonance, nasality, intelligibility), need for secondary speech surgery, and complications. A recent systematic review compared the outcomes of cleft palate repair using the Furlow technique and straight-line repair methods with IVV[103] (Level II evidence). The straight-line techniques include the von Langenbeck, V-Y pushback, and 2-flap palatoplasty. Ponduri and colleagues[103] reviewed data from 11 retrospective studies and 1 prospective randomized trial.

They found an oronasal fistula rate of 7.87% in the group receiving the Furlow repair and 9.81% in the straight-line with IVV group. Children with more severe clefting as determined by the Veau classification were more likely to develop a fistula. The rate of fistula formation in the Furlow and straight-line groups was not significantly different.

Velopharyngeal insufficiency was determined by the need for secondary corrective surgery. The difference in secondary surgery rates between the Furlow and straight-line groups was significantly different only in the unilateral cleft lip and palate population. In the Furlow group, between 0% and 11.4% of patients with an isolated cleft palate and between 0% and 6.7% with unilateral cleft lip and palate underwent secondary surgery. In the straight-line IVV group, between 9.1% and 29.2% of those with an isolated cleft palate and between 6.7% and 19.4% of those with unilateral cleft lip and palate underwent secondary surgery. Overall, the Furlow technique may be the preferred technique, as it leads to a decreased rate of secondary surgery[104] (Level II evidence).

Complications and Concerns

Oronasal fistula

The development of oronasal fistula is a concern following cleft palate repair, especially if the closure is under tension. An overall fistula rate of 4.9% has been reported[105] (Level II evidence). The most common location of occurrence is at the soft and hard palate junction. Using techniques that reduce closure tension, such as the hamular release and relaxing incisions, may decrease fistula occurrence. There are some reports purporting the benefit of placing a layer of decellularized dermis in the palatal closure, as an interpositional graft that may reduce the fistula rate. In a retrospective review of 31 cleft palate cases repaired using the Furlow technique and decellularized dermis, only 1 patient developed a fistula postoperatively[78] (Level IV evidence). This small cohort was not compared with another similar group. In another retrospective review of 7 patients, a 2-flap approach with IVV was used for primary repair[106] (Level IV evidence). Decellularized dermal grafts were used in the repair and there were no fistulas. Prospective studies would be needed to develop the evidence that decellularized dermis has a role in primary palate repairs for decreasing the risk of fistula occurrence. Additional cost and risk of viral transmission are major detractors to the routine use of acellular cadaveric dermis in cleft palate repair.

Velopharyngeal insufficiency

Velopharyngeal dysfunction after primary cleft palate repair may require secondary speech surgery with rates reported from 5% to 38%.[107] The inability to close the velopharyngeal sphincter leads to nasal air escape during speech. The resulting hypernasality can lead the child to develop compensatory speech errors (eg, glottal stops) and speech quality suffers.[108] Treatment for velopharyngeal insufficiency (VPI) involves secondary speech therapy and correction, either surgical or nonsurgical. Nonsurgical treatment includes an oropharyngeal obturator, prosthetic, or palatal lift; however, their use is limited by poor patient tolerance.

There are 4 components of the velopharynx: the soft palate anteriorly, the lateral pharyngeal walls bilaterally, and the posterior pharyngeal wall posteriorly. Surgery to restore velopharyngeal competence can involve each of these components; however, the most common procedures are the pharyngeal flap and sphincter pharyngoplasty (**Fig. 9**). Retrospective studies have not demonstrated the superiority of one procedure in terms of VPI resolution and postoperative complications[109,110] (Level IV evidence). The speech outcomes (eg, nasal air emissions and resonance scores) of pharyngeal flap surgery were reported in a recent retrospective study of 61 patients. Speech scores increased in all patients with a surgical revision rate of 19.7% (comparable to previously published studies).[111] The difficulty in comparing outcomes from secondary speech surgery lies in the lack of consistent reporting methods, thus supporting evidence that cleft centers should encourage consistent documentation, which would foster interdisciplinary and multi-institutional studies.

Two prospective randomized trials were performed to compare the pharyngeal flap and sphincter pharyngoplasty operations. Neither study found a significant difference between the 2 in terms of VPI outcomes or complications[112,113] (Level I evidence). To optimize outcomes, the width of the pharyngeal flap or the lateral flaps in a sphincter pharyngoplasty can be customized according to the size of the velopharyngeal gap and the quality of palatal and lateral wall motions[114] (Level I evidence).

GENERAL THERAPEUTIC CONSIDERATIONS FOR CLEFT LIP AND PALATE
Airway Concerns

Children who have cleft palate are at a higher risk of upper airway obstruction. Studies have found the incidence of airway obstruction to be up to 18% in nonsyndromic children with an isolated cleft palate[115,116] (Levels II and IV evidence). The risk increases even more when the cleft anomaly occurs as part of a syndrome. In the postoperative period, this risk increases. There are a few contributors to airway obstruction postoperatively. First, closure of the cleft causes a decrease in available airway space. Second, prolonged tongue

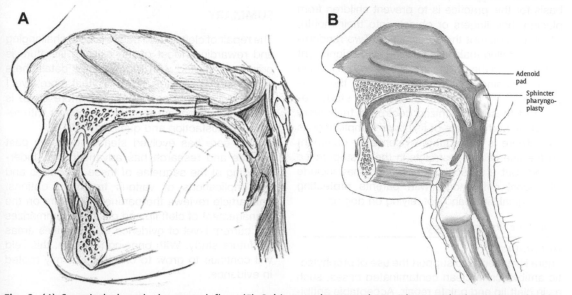

Fig. 9. (*A*) Superiorly based pharyngeal flap. (*B*) Sphincter pharyngoplasty. Along with the Furlow double-opposing Z-plasty (see **Fig. 7**), these represent the most common secondary speech surgeries to address velopharyngeal insufficiency after cleft palate repair. (*From* [A] Willging JP, Cohen AP. Pharyngeal flap surgery. In: Goudy S, Tollefson TT, editors. Complete cleft care. New York: Thieme; 2015. p. 173, with permission; and [B] Boss EF, Sie K. Sphincter pharyngoplasty. In: Goudy S, Tollefson TT, editors. Complete cleft care. New York: Thieme; 2015. p. 178, with permission.)

retraction during the procedure can cause acute swelling. In anticipation of potential postoperative airway obstruction, a nasal airway can be placed before extubation to decrease the risks of airway compromise.

Feeding

There is no consensus on postoperative feeding protocols following repair of cleft lip and/or palate. The World Health Organization recommends exclusive breastfeeding until 6 months of age, and a recent Cochrane systematic review found a weakly positive effect of breastfeeding on postoperative weight gain compared with spoon feeding in infants with cleft lip[117] (Level I evidence). Mothers should therefore be encouraged to breastfeed when possible, but breast milk pumping and use of a cleft feeder, such as the Haberman, Pigeon, Mead Johnson, or others. In the same review, there was insufficient evidence to conclude whether squeezable bottles are beneficial compared with rigid feeding bottles for improving growth and development.[117] However, a squeezable bottle may be preferred for ease of use in infants with cleft anomalies. Finally, maxillary appliances did not have an adverse effect on growth.[117]

Arm Restraints

Most cleft surgeons in the United States use arm restraints during the postoperative period.[118] The basis for this practice is to prevent children from placing their fingers or objects into their mouth, which can disrupt the surgical site. Two randomized controlled trials failed to show any significant differences in the development of oronasal fistulae in the restrained group compared with the unrestrained[119,120] (Level I evidence). The study designs of these randomized controlled trials were not ideal, and the rate of fistula or complication is rare. There is inadequate evidence to comment on the use of arm restraints in the postoperative period, but a reasonable approach may include situational differences, with parents protecting the surgical sites, and not relying on dogma.

Relevant Pharmacology

Antibiotics

There is evidence to support the use of prophylactic antibiotics in clean contaminated cases, such as in cleft lip and palate repair. Acceptable antibiotics include cefazolin and clindamycin. Antibiotics should be administered before the surgical incision is made. There is no evidence for ongoing antibiotics following surgery[121] (Levels I and IV evidence).

Steroids

Perioperative dexamethasone may decrease the risk of airway swelling and subsequent respiratory distress without detrimental effects on wound healing[115,116] (Levels II and IV evidence).

Analgesia

For immediate postoperative pain control, an infraorbital nerve block with longer-acting local anesthetics, such as bupivacaine or ropivacaine, can be used[122] (Level III evidence). Much of the evidence on post–head and neck surgery analgesia in children is based on the tonsillectomy literature. With the exception of ketorolac, nonsteroidal anti-inflammatory drugs have not been associated with an increased risk of bleeding complications[123–125] (Levels I and IV evidence). Codeine has recently fallen out of favor. Genetic polymorphisms render some individuals unable to metabolize codeine to morphine, whereas others will hypermetabolize it[126,127] (Levels I and II evidence). Overall, codeine has not been found to be more effective at controlling pain compared with plain acetaminophen after tonsillectomy[128] (Level II evidence). Furthermore, hypermetabolism of codeine can lead to toxic levels of morphine and has been associated with postoperative mortality[126] (Level IV evidence). For these reasons, a regimen consisting of acetaminophen and ibuprofen may be the best option, taking into account the potential risk of bleeding with nonsteroidal anti-inflammatory drugs.

SUMMARY

The repair of cleft lip and palate is both challenging and rewarding. Most of the existing literature is practice-centered with retrospective data. There is growing recognition, however, that more level I and II evidence is needed. Furthermore, there is a shift toward patient-reported outcomes with regard to satisfaction and quality of life.

Cleft care has evolved steadily over the past decade and research has advanced our understanding of the sequelae of these anomalies and the implications of various treatment options. This article reviews the pertinent literature on the management of cleft lip and palate. It summarizes the current level of evidence and identifies areas for future study. With ongoing research, this field will continue to grow to one that is firmly rooted in evidence.

REFERENCES

1. Canfield MA, Honein MA, Yuskiv N, et al. National estimates and race/ethnic-specific variation of selected birth defects in the United States,

1999-2001. Birth Defects Res A Clin Mol Teratol 2006;76(11):747–56.

2. Tollefson TT, Sykes JM. Unilateral cleft lip. In: Goudy SG, Tollefson TT, editors. Complete cleft care. New York: Thieme; 2014. p. 37–59.

3. Sitzman TJ, Girotto JA, Marcus JR. Current surgical practices in cleft care: unilateral cleft lip repair. Plast Reconstr Surg 2008;121(5):261e–70e.

4. Holtmann B, Wray RC. A randomized comparison of triangular and rotation-advancement unilateral cleft lip repairs. Plast Reconstr Surg 1983;71(2):172–9.

5. Randall P, Whitaker LA, LaRossa D. The importance of muscle reconstruction in primary and secondary cleft lip repair. Plast Reconstr Surg 1974; 54(3):316–23.

6. Chowdri NA, Darzi MA, Ashraf MM. A comparative study of surgical results with rotation-advancement and triangular flap techniques in unilateral cleft lip. Br J Plast Surg 1990;43(5):551–6.

7. Manchester WM. The repair of double cleft lip as part of an integrated program. Plast Reconstr Surg 1970;45(3):207–16.

8. Nagase T, Januszkiewicz JS, Keall HJ, et al. The effect of muscle repair on postoperative facial skeletal growth in children with bilateral cleft lip and palate. Scand J Plast Reconstr Surg Hand Surg 1998;32(4):395–405.

9. Delaire J. Theoretical principles and technique of functional closure of the lip and nasal aperture. J Maxillofac Surg 1978;6(2):109–16.

10. Joos U. Skeletal growth after muscular reconstruction for cleft lip, alveolus and palate. Br J Oral Maxillofac Surg 1995;33(3):139–44.

11. Markus AF, Precious DS. Effect of primary surgery for cleft lip and palate on mid-facial growth. Br J Oral Maxillofac Surg 1997;35(1):6–10.

12. Chen PK, Noordhoff MS, Liou EJ. Treatment of complete bilateral cleft lip-nasal deformity. Semin Plast Surg 2005;19(4):329–41.

13. Matsuo K, Hirose T. Preoperative non-surgical overcorrection of cleft lip nasal deformity. Br J Plast Surg 1991;44(1):5–11.

14. Grayson BH, Cutting CB. Presurgical nasoalveolar orthopedic molding in primary correction of the nose, lip, and alveolus of infants born with unilateral and bilateral clefts. Cleft Palate Craniofac J 2001;38(3):193–8.

15. Mulliken JB. Primary repair of bilateral cleft lip and nasal deformity. Plast Reconstr Surg 2001;108(1): 181–94 [examination: 195–6].

16. Xu H, Salyer KE, Genecov ER. Primary bilateral one-stage cleft lip/nose repair: 40-year Dallas experience: part I. J Craniofac Surg 2009; 20(Suppl 2):1913–26.

17. Tan SP, Greene AK, Mulliken JB. Current surgical management of bilateral cleft lip in North America. Plast Reconstr Surg 2012;129(6):1347–55.

18. Aburezq H, Daskalogiannakis J, Forrest C. Management of the prominent premaxilla in bilateral cleft lip and palate. Cleft Palate Craniofac J 2006; 43(1):92–5.

19. Shaye D. Update on outcomes research for cleft lip and palate. Curr Opin Otolaryngol Head Neck Surg 2014;22(4):255–9.

20. Campbell A, Costello BJ, Ruiz RL. Cleft lip and palate surgery: an update of clinical outcomes for primary repair. Oral Maxillofac Surg Clin North Am 2010;22(1):43–58.

21. Hallock GG. In utero cleft lip repair in A/J mice. Plast Reconstr Surg 1985;75(6):785–90.

22. Longaker MT, Stern M, Lorenz P, et al. A model for fetal cleft lip repair in lambs. Plast Reconstr Surg 1992;90(5):750–6.

23. Slade P, Emerson DJ, Freedlander E. A longitudinal comparison of the psychological impact on mothers of neonatal and 3 month repair of cleft lip. Br J Plast Surg 1999;52(1):1–5.

24. Cladis F, Damian D. Anesthesia for cleft patients. In: Kirschner RE, Losee JE, editors. Comprehensive cleft care. New York: McGraw-Hill; 2009. p. 211–21.

25. Wilhelmsen HR, Musgrave RH. Complications of cleft lip surgery. Cleft Palate J 1966;3:223–31.

26. Shaw WC, Brattström V, Mølsted K, et al. The Eurocleft study: intercenter study of the treatment outcome in patients with complete cleft lip and palate. Part 5: discussion and conclusions. Cleft Palate Craniofac J 2005;42:93–8.

27. Uzel A, Alparslan ZN. Long-term effects of presurgical infant orthopedics in patients with cleft lip and palate: a systematic review. Cleft Palate Craniofac J 2011;48(5):587–95.

28. de Ladeira PR, Alonso N. Protocols in cleft lip and palate treatment: systematic review. Plast Surg Int 2012;2012:562892.

29. Barillas I, Dec W, Warren SM, et al. Nasoalveolar molding improves long-term nasal symmetry in complete unilateral cleft lip-cleft palate patients. Plast Reconstr Surg 2009;123(3):1002–6.

30. Lee CT, Garfinkle JS, Warren SM, et al. Nasoalveolar molding improves appearance of children with bilateral cleft lip-cleft palate. Plast Reconstr Surg 2008;122(4):1131–7.

31. Liou EJ, Subramanian M, Chen PK. Progressive changes of columella length and nasal growth after nasoalveolar molding in bilateral cleft patients: a 3-year follow-up study. Plast Reconstr Surg 2007; 119(2):642–8.

32. Liou EJ, Subramanian M, Chen PK, et al. The progressive changes of nasal symmetry and growth after nasoalveolar molding: a three-year follow-up study. Plast Reconstr Surg 2004;114(4):858–64.

33. Abbott MM, Meara JG. Nasoalveolar molding in cleft care: is it efficacious? Plast Reconstr Surg 2012;130(3):659–66.

34. Sischo L, Chan JW, Stein M, et al. Nasoalveolar molding: prevalence of cleft centers offering NAM and who seeks it. Cleft Palate Craniofac J 2012; 49(3):270–5.

35. Randall P. A lip adhesion operation in cleft lip surgery. Plast Reconstr Surg 1965;35:371–6.

36. Hamilton R, Graham WP 3rd, Randall P. The role of the lip adhesion procedure in cleft lip repair. Cleft Palate J 1971;8:1–9.

37. Salyer KE, Genecov ER, Genecov DG. Unilateral cleft lip-nose repair: a 33-year experience. J Craniofac Surg 2003;14(4):549–58.

38. Enemark H, Sindet-Pedersen S, Bundgaard M. Long-term results after secondary bone grafting of alveolar clefts. J Oral Maxillofac Surg 1987; 45(11):913–9.

39. Trindade-Suedam IK, da Silva Filho OG, Carvalho RM, et al. Timing of alveolar bone grafting determines different outcomes in patients with unilateral cleft palate. J Craniofac Surg 2012;23(5): 1283–6.

40. Eppley BL. Alveolar cleft bone grafting (Part I): primary bone grafting. J Oral Maxillofac Surg 1996; 54(1):74–82.

41. Tollefson TT, Senders CW, Sykes JM. Changing perspectives in cleft lip and palate: from acrylic to allele. Arch Facial Plast Surg 2008;10(6):395–400.

42. Guyuron B. MOC-PS(SM) CME article: late cleft lip nasal deformity. Plast Reconstr Surg 2008;121(4 Suppl):1–11.

43. Broadbent TR, Woolf RM. Cleft lip nasal deformity. Ann Plast Surg 1984;12(3):216–34.

44. Anastassov GE, Joos U, Zollner B. Evaluation of the results of delayed rhinoplasty in cleft lip and palate patients. Functional and aesthetic implications and factors that affect successful nasal repair. Br J Oral Maxillofac Surg 1998;36(6):416–24.

45. McComb H. Treatment of the unilateral cleft lip nose. Plast Reconstr Surg 1975;55(5):596–601.

46. McComb H. Primary correction of unilateral cleft lip nasal deformity: a 10-year review. Plast Reconstr Surg 1985;75(6):791–9.

47. McComb HK, Coghlan BA. Primary repair of the unilateral cleft lip nose: completion of a longitudinal study. Cleft Palate Craniofac J 1996;33(1):23–30 [discussion: 30–1].

48. Anastassov GE, Joos U. Comprehensive management of cleft lip and palate deformities. J Oral Maxillofac Surg 2001;59(9):1062–75 [discussion: 1075–7].

49. Anderl H, Hussl H, Ninkovic M. Primary simultaneous lip and nose repair in the unilateral cleft lip and palate. Plast Reconstr Surg 2008;121(3):959–70.

50. Brussé CA, Van der Werff JF, Stevens HP, et al. Symmetry and morbidity assessment of unilateral complete cleft lip nose corrected with or without primary nasal correction. Cleft Palate Craniofac J 1999;36(4):361–6.

51. Wolfe SA. A pastiche for the cleft lip nose. Plast Reconstr Surg 2004;114(1):1–9.

52. Salyer KE. Excellence in cleft lip and palate treatment. J Craniofac Surg 2001;12(1):2–5.

53. Byrd HS, Salomon J. Primary correction of the unilateral cleft nasal deformity. Plast Reconstr Surg 2000;106(6):1276–86.

54. Wong GB, Burvin R, Mulliken JB. Resorbable internal splint: an adjunct to primary correction of unilateral cleft lip-nasal deformity. Plast Reconstr Surg 2002;110(2):385–91.

55. Cenzi R, Guarda L. A dynamic nostril splint in the surgery of the nasal tip: technical innovation. J Craniomaxillofac Surg 1996;24(2):88–91.

56. Nakajima T, Yoshimura Y, Sakakibara A. Augmentation of the nostril splint for retaining the corrected contour of the cleft lip nose. Plast Reconstr Surg 1990;85(2):182–6.

57. Sharma VP, Bella H, Cadier MM, et al. Outcomes in facial aesthetics in cleft lip and palate surgery: a systematic review. J Plast Reconstr Aesthet Surg 2012;65(9):1233–45.

58. Mulliken JB, Wu JK, Padwa BL. Repair of bilateral cleft lip: review, revisions, and reflections. J Craniofac Surg 2003;14(5):609–20.

59. Semb G, Brattström V, Mølsted K, et al. The Eurocleft study: intercenter study of treatment outcome in patients with complete cleft lip and palate. Part 1: introduction and treatment experience. Cleft Palate Craniofac J 2005;42(1):64–8.

60. Mehrotra D, Pradhan R. Cleft lip: our experience in repair. J Maxillofac Oral Surg 2010;9(1):60–3.

61. Schonmeyr B, Wendby L, Campbell A. Early surgical complications after primary cleft lip repair: a report of 3108 consecutive cases. Cleft Palate Craniofac J 2014. [Epub ahead of print].

62. Nagy K, Mommaerts MY. Postoperative wound management after cleft lip surgery. Cleft Palate Craniofac J 2011;48(5):584–6.

63. Bardach J. The influence of cleft lip repair on facial growth. Cleft Palate J 1990;27(1):76–8.

64. Bardach J, Mooney MP. The relationship between lip pressure following lip repair and craniofacial growth: an experimental study in beagles. Plast Reconstr Surg 1984;73(4):544–55.

65. Bishara SE, de Arrendondo RS, Vales HP, et al. Dentofacial relationships in persons with unoperated clefts: comparisons between three cleft types. Am J Orthod 1985;87(6):481–507.

66. Honda Y, Suzuki A, Nakamura N, et al. Relationship between primary palatal form and maxillofacial growth in Japanese children with unilateral cleft lip and palate: infancy to adolescence. Cleft Palate Craniofac J 2002;39(5):527–34.

67. Li Y, Shi B, Song QG, et al. Effects of lip repair on maxillary growth and facial soft tissue development in patients with a complete unilateral cleft of lip,

alveolus and palate. J Craniomaxillofac Surg 2006; 34(6):355–61.

68. Rousseau P, Metzger M, Frucht S, et al. Effect of lip closure on early maxillary growth in patients with cleft lip and palate. JAMA Facial Plast Surg 2013; 15(5):369–73.

69. Huang MH, Lee ST, Rajendran K. A fresh cadaveric study of the paratubal muscles: implications for eustachian tube function in cleft palate. Plast Reconstr Surg 1997;100(4):833–42.

70. Shaw WC, Semb G, Nelson P, et al. The Eurocleft project 1996-2000: overview. J Craniomaxillofac Surg 2001;29(3):131–40 [discussion: 141–2].

71. Bardach J. Two-flap palatoplasty: Bardach's technique. Oper Tech Plast Reconstr Surg 1995;2:211.

72. Marsh JL, Galic M. Maxillofacial osteotomies for patients with cleft lip and palate. Clin Plast Surg 1989;16(4):803–14.

73. Andrades P, Espinosa-de-los-Monteros A, Shell DH 4th, et al. The importance of radical intravelar veloplasty during two-flap palatoplasty. Plast Reconstr Surg 2008;122(4):1121–30.

74. Sommerlad BC, Mehendale FV, Birch MJ, et al. Palate re-repair revisited. Cleft Palate Craniofac J 2002;39(3):295–307.

75. Hassan ME, Askar S. Does palatal muscle reconstruction affect the functional outcome of cleft palate surgery? Plast Reconstr Surg 2007;119(6): 1859–65.

76. Williams WN, Seagle MB, Pegoraro-Krook MI, et al. Prospective clinical trial comparing outcome measures between Furlow and von Langenbeck palatoplasties for UCLP. Ann Plast Surg 2011;66(2):154–63.

77. Steele MH, Seagle MB. Palatal fistula repair using acellular dermal matrix: the University of Florida experience. Ann Plast Surg 2006;56(1):50–3 [discussion: 53].

78. Helling ER, Dev VR, Garza J, et al. Low fistula rate in palatal clefts closed with the Furlow technique using decellularized dermis. Plast Reconstr Surg 2006;117(7):2361–5.

79. Kirschner RE, Wang P, Jawad AF, et al. Cleft-palate repair by modified Furlow double-opposing Z-plasty: the Children's Hospital of Philadelphia experience. Plast Reconstr Surg 1999;104(7): 1998–2010 [discussion: 2011–4].

80. Yu CC, Chen PK, Chen YR. Comparison of speech results after Furlow palatoplasty and von Langenbeck palatoplasty in incomplete cleft of the secondary palate. Chang Gung Med J 2001;24(10):628–32.

81. Gunther E, Wisser JR, Cohen MA, et al. Palatoplasty: Furlow's double reversing Z-plasty versus intravelar veloplasty. Cleft Palate Craniofac J 1998;35(6):546–9.

82. Hardin-Jones MA, Jones DL. Speech production of preschoolers with cleft palate. Cleft Palate Craniofac J 2005;42(1):7–13.

83. Dorf DS, Curtin JW. Early cleft palate repair and speech outcome. Plast Reconstr Surg 1982;70(1): 74–81.

84. Pradel W, Senf D, Mai R, et al. One-stage palate repair improves speech outcome and early maxillary growth in patients with cleft lip and palate. J Physiol Pharmacol 2009;60(Suppl 8):37–41.

85. Chapman KL, Hardin-Jones MA, Goldstein JA, et al. Timing of palatal surgery and speech outcome. Cleft Palate Craniofac J 2008;45(3):297–308.

86. Kim T, Ishikawa H, Chu S, et al. Constriction of the maxillary dental arch by mucoperiosteal denudation of the palate. Cleft Palate Craniofac J 2002; 39(4):425–31.

87. Liao YF, Cole TJ, Mars M. Hard palate repair timing and facial growth in unilateral cleft lip and palate: a longitudinal study. Cleft Palate Craniofac J 2006; 43(5):547–56.

88. Chen ZQ, Qian YF, Wang GM, et al. Sagittal maxillary growth in patients with unoperated isolated cleft palate. Cleft Palate Craniofac J 2009;46(6): 664–7.

89. Ye B, Ruan C, Hu J, et al. A comparative study on dental-arch morphology in adult unoperated and operated cleft palate patients. J Craniofac Surg 2010;21(3):811–5.

90. Lilja J, Mars M, Elander A, et al. Analysis of dental arch relationships in Swedish unilateral cleft lip and palate subjects: 20-year longitudinal consecutive series treated with delayed hard palate closure. Cleft Palate Craniofac J 2006;43(5):606–11.

91. Mølsted K, Brattström V, Prahl-Andersen B, et al. The Eurocleft study: intercenter study of treatment outcome in patients with complete cleft lip and palate. Part 3: dental arch relationships. Cleft Palate Craniofac J 2005;42(1):78–82.

92. Markus AF, Delaire J, Smith WP. Facial balance in cleft lip and palate. II. Cleft lip and palate and secondary deformities. Br J Oral Maxillofac Surg 1992; 30(5):296–304.

93. Liao YF, Yang IY, Wang R, et al. Two-stage palate repair with delayed hard palate closure is related to favorable maxillary growth in unilateral cleft lip and palate. Plast Reconstr Surg 2010;125(5): 1503–10.

94. Ross RB. Treatment variables affecting facial growth in complete unilateral cleft lip and palate. Cleft Palate J 1987;24(1):5–77.

95. Bardach J, Morris HL, Olin WH. Late results of primary veloplasty: the Marburg Project. Plast Reconstr Surg 1984;73(2):207–18.

96. Schweckendiek W, Doz P. Primary veloplasty: long-term results without maxillary deformity. a twenty-five year report. Cleft Palate J 1978;15(3):268–74.

97. Fara M, Brousilova M. Experiences with early closure of velum and later closure of hard palate. Plast Reconstr Surg 1969;44(2):134–41.

98. Kirschner RE, Randall P, Wang P, et al. Cleft palate repair at 3 to 7 months of age. Plast Reconstr Surg 2000;105(6):2127–32.

99. Cho BC, Kim JY, Yang JD, et al. Influence of the Furlow palatoplasty for patients with submucous cleft palate on facial growth. J Craniofac Surg 2004;15(4):547–54 [discussion: 555].

100. Bluestone CD, Beery QC, Cantekin EI, et al. Eustachian tube ventilatory function in relation to cleft palate. Ann Otol Rhinol Laryngol 1975;84(3 Pt 1):333–8.

101. Fria TJ, Paradise JL, Sabo DL, et al. Conductive hearing loss in infants and young children with cleft palate. J Pediatr 1987;111(1):84–7.

102. Klockars T, Rautio J. Early placement of ventilation tubes in cleft lip and palate patients: does palatal closure affect tube occlusion and short-term outcome? Int J Pediatr Otorhinolaryngol 2012; 76(10):1481–4.

103. Ponduri S, Bradley R, Ellis PE, et al. The management of otitis media with early routine insertion of grommets in children with cleft palate–a systematic review. Cleft Palate Craniofac J 2009;46(1):30–8.

104. Timbang MR, Gharb BB, Rampazzo A, et al. A systematic review comparing Furlow double-opposing Z-plasty and straight-line intravelar velo-plasty methods of cleft palate repair. Plast Reconstr Surg 2014;134(5):1014–22.

105. Bykowski MR, Naran S, Winger DG, et al. The rate of oronasal fistula following primary cleft palate surgery: a meta-analysis. Cleft Palate Craniofac J 2014. [Epub ahead of print].

106. Clark JM, Saffold SH, Israel JM. Decellularized dermal grafting in cleft palate repair. Arch Facial Plast Surg 2003;5(1):40–4 [discussion: 45].

107. Witt PD, D'Antonio LL. Velopharyngeal insufficiency and secondary palatal management. A new look at an old problem. Clin Plast Surg 1993;20(4):707–21.

108. Fisher DM, Sommerlad BC. Cleft lip, cleft palate, and velopharyngeal insufficiency. Plast Reconstr Surg 2011;128(4):342e–60e.

109. de Serres LM, Deleyiannis FW, Eblen LE, et al. Results with sphincter pharyngoplasty and pharyngeal flap. Int J Pediatr Otorhinolaryngol 1999;48(1):17–25.

110. Pensler JM, Reich DS. A comparison of speech results after the pharyngeal flap and the dynamic sphincteroplasty procedures. Ann Plast Surg 1991;26(5):441–3.

111. Setabutr D, Roth CT, Nolen DD, et al. Pharyngeal flap for velopharyngeal insufficiency: revision rates and speech outcomes. JAMA Facial Plast Surg 2015. http://dx.doi.org/10.1001/jamafacial.2015. 0093.

112. Abyholm F, D'Antonio L, Davidson Ward SL, et al. Pharyngeal flap and sphincterplasty for velopharyngeal insufficiency have equal outcome at 1 year postoperatively: results of a randomized trial. Cleft Palate Craniofac J 2005;42(5):501–11.

113. Ysunza A, Pamplona MC, Molina F, et al. Surgery for speech in cleft palate patients. Int J Pediatr Otorhinolaryngol 2004;68(12):1499–505.

114. Ysunza A, Pamplona C, Ramírez E, et al. Velopharyngeal surgery: a prospective randomized study of pharyngeal flaps and sphincter pharyngoplasties. Plast Reconstr Surg 2002;110(6):1401–7.

115. Senders CW, Di Mauro SM, Brodie HA, et al. The efficacy of perioperative steroid therapy in pediatric primary palatoplasty. Cleft Palate Craniofac J 1999;36(4):340–4.

116. Antony AK, Sloan GM. Airway obstruction following palatoplasty: analysis of 247 consecutive operations. Cleft Palate Craniofac J 2002;39(2):145–8.

117. Bessell A, Hooper L, Shaw WC, et al. Feeding interventions for growth and development in infants with cleft lip, cleft palate or cleft lip and palate. Cochrane Database Syst Rev 2011;(2):CD003315.

118. Katzel EB, Basile P, Koltz PF, et al. Current surgical practices in cleft care: cleft palate repair techniques and postoperative care. Plast Reconstr Surg 2009;124(3):899–906.

119. Jigjinni V, Kangesu T, Sommerlad BC. Do babies require arm splints after cleft palate repair? Br J Plast Surg 1993;46(8):681–5.

120. Huth J, Petersen D, Lehman JA. The use of postoperative restraints in children after cleft lip or cleft palate repair: a preliminary report. ISRN Plastic Surgery 2013;2013:3.

121. Russell MD, Goldberg AN. What is the evidence for use of antibiotic prophylaxis in clean-contaminated head and neck surgery? Laryngoscope 2012;122(5):945–6.

122. Liau JY, Sadove AM, van Aalst JA. An evidence-based approach to cleft palate repair. Plast Reconstr Surg 2010;126(6):2216–21.

123. Cardwell M, Siviter G, Smith A. Non-steroidal anti-inflammatory drugs and perioperative bleeding in paediatric tonsillectomy. Cochrane Database Syst Rev 2005;(2):CD003591.

124. Judkins JH, Dray TG, Hubbell RN. Intraoperative ketorolac and posttonsillectomy bleeding. Arch Otolaryngol Head Neck Surg 1996;122(9):937–40.

125. Bailey R, Sinha C, Burgess LP. Ketorolac tromethamine and hemorrhage in tonsillectomy: a prospective, randomized, double-blind study. Laryngoscope 1997;107(2):166–9.

126. Ciszkowski C, Madadi P, Phillips MS, et al. Codeine, ultrarapid-metabolism genotype, and postoperative death. N Engl J Med 2009;361(8):827–8.

127. Williams DG, Patel A, Howard RF. Pharmacogenetics of codeine metabolism in an urban population of children and its implications for analgesic reliability. Br J Anaesth 2002;89(6):839–45.

128. Baugh RF, Archer SM, Mitchell RB, et al. Clinical practice guideline: tonsillectomy in children. Otolaryngol Head Neck Surg 2011;144(1 Suppl):S1–30.

Evidence-Based Medicine in the Treatment of Infantile Hemangiomas

Robert G. Keller, MD[a], Krishna G. Patel, MD, PhD[b],*

KEYWORDS

- Vascular anomalies • Infantile hemangioma • Propranolol therapy • Steroid therapy
- Pulsed dye laser therapy

KEY POINTS

- The International Society for the Study of Vascular Anomalies (ISSVA) (www.issva.org) is the presiding organization for the classification of vascular anomalies.
- Oral steroids are now considered a second choice option for the management of infantile hemangiomas (IHs).
- Oral propranolol is becoming the first line of treatment of the management of IHs if observation or laser therapy is not sufficient.
- Surgery has become more accepted as a means of early treatment of hemangiomas and relies on a physician's clinical judgment regarding timing of intervention.
- Multimodality algorithms, specifically addressing individual components of these tumors, result in the best functional and cosmetic outcomes.

HISTORICAL PERSPECTIVE AND CURRENT CLASSIFICATION SCHEME

The broader picture of vascular anomalies must first be elucidated to better understand the disease process of hemangiomas. The history of facial vascular anomalies is one plagued by confusing nomenclature, misdiagnosis, and lack of a unified consensus on the classification of an incredibly broad group of lesions. In 1982, however, the diligent work of Mulliken and Glowacki[1] introduced the first classification system of vascular anomalies. Their study analyzed cellular characteristics of 49 vascular lesions and distinguished vascular tumors from vascular malformations based on histopathology, increased endothelial cell turnover, and differences in clinical history.[1] A decade later, the ISSVA was founded and has since led the way in maintaining international consensus on the classification of vascular anomalies.[2] The classification system has enhanced physician understanding and ability to accurately diagnose and appropriately prescribe therapy in patients afflicted with vascular anomalies.

The current classification scheme for vascular anomalies undergoes frequent updating and redefining by ISSVA (**Table 1**). Currently, IH is classified as a benign vascular tumor. Like all vascular tumors/hemangiomas, IHs are characterized by increased endothelial cell turnover, which differentiates them from vascular malformations.[1] Current theories surrounding the pathophysiology of IHs revolve around its unique expression of glucose transporter protein 1 (GLUT-1), possibly

Disclosures: None of the authors has a financial interest in any of the products, devices, or drugs mentioned in this article.
[a] Department of Otolaryngology – Head and Neck Surgery, Medical University of South Carolina, 135 Rutledge Avenue, Charleston, SC 29425, USA; [b] Facial Plastic and Reconstructive Surgery, Department of Otolaryngology – Head and Neck Surgery, Medical University of South Carolina, 135 Rutledge Avenue, Charleston, SC 29425, USA
* Corresponding author.
E-mail address: krishnapatel72@gmail.com

Facial Plast Surg Clin N Am 23 (2015) 373–392
http://dx.doi.org/10.1016/j.fsc.2015.04.009
1064-7406/15/$ – see front matter © 2015 Elsevier Inc. All rights reserved.

Table 1
International Society for the Study of Vascular Anomalies classification for vascular anomalies

	Vascular Anomalies			
		Vascular Malformations		
Vascular Tumors	Simple	Combined	Of Major Named Vessels	Associated with Other Anomalies
Benign vascular tumors IH Congenital hemangioma Rapidly involuting congenital hemangioma[a] Noninvoluting congenital hemangioma Partially involuting congenital hemangioma Tufted angioma Spindle-cell hemangioma Epithelioid hemangioma Pyogenic granuloma (also known as lobular C hemangioma) Others Locally aggressive or borderline vascular tumors Kaposiform hemangioendothelioma Retiform hemangioendothelioma Papillary intralymphatic angioendothelioma, Dabska tumor Composite hemangioendothelioma Kaposi sarcoma Others Malignant vascular tumors Angiosarcoma Epithelioid hemangioendothelioma Others	C malformations L malformations V malformations AV Ms[a] AV fistula[a]	Defined as 2 or more vascular malformations identified in 1 lesion. Can be composed of any combination of: C, L, V, AV[a]	Channel-type or truncal malformations	Klippel-Trénaunay syndrome Parkes Weber syndrome Servelle-Martorell syndrome Sturge-Weber syndrome Limb CM + limb hypertrophy Maffucci syndrome Macrocephaly–CM Microcephaly–CM CLOVES syndrome Proteus syndrome Bannayan-Riley-Ruvalcaba syndrome

Abbreviations: AV, arteriovenous; C, capillary; CLOVES, congenital, lipomatous, overgrowth, vascular malformations, epidermal nevi, and spinal/skeletal anomalies and/or scoliosis; CM, capillary malformation; L, lymphatic; M, malformation; V, venous.

[a] High-flow lesions.

suggesting origin from placental endothelium, which is the only other cell in the body that expresses GLUT-1.[3,4] The unique expression of GLUT-1 in IHs makes it an important marker for histologic diagnosis. IHs have been subclassified based on their diverse range of presentations. They are categorized based on depth of tissue involvement, including superficial, compound (mixed-type), and deep and reticular hemangiomas as well as by their patterns of distribution as either focal, multifocal, segmental, or indeterminate (**Table 2**). Subclassification of these lesions is imperative to make appropriate treatment decisions.

As evidence-based medicine has become the modern-day norm, it is now understood as the duty of the physicians to incorporate such evidence in their everyday practice and decision making. In treating facial vascular tumors, a host of therapeutic modalities exists, all with different levels of evidence supporting their efficacy, safety profiles, and utilization algorithms. This study attempts to shed light on the state of the current evidence supporting different treatment modalities for IHs.

EPIDEMIOLOGY AND CLINICAL PRESENTATION

IHs are the most common benign vascular tumors of infancy and childhood, occurring in 4.5% of all infants by age 3 months and in up to 12% by 1 year of age.[5,6] IHs occur between 3 and 6 times more frequently in girls than boys; are seen more often in whites, premature infants, and twins; and tend to afflict offspring of mothers of higher maternal age.[5,7,8] Approximately 60% of these occur in the head and neck region, 25% on the trunk and 15% on the extremities.[9] At birth, most IHs are absent or have a small premonitory mark, such as a pale macule.[10] By 1 to 4 weeks of age, most IHs have become clinically apparent. Depending on depth of involvement, IHs have a diverse appearance; superficial IHs tend to be bright red, slightly elevated, noncompressible plaques, whereas deep IHs are soft, warm, and bluish in color.[11] Compound hemangiomas develop both deep and superficial components (**Fig. 1**). Focal and multifocal lesions present in 1 or multiple locations, respectively, whereas segmental hemangiomas pattern within facial dermatomes.[12,13] Segmental hemangiomas are classically associated with PHACE (association of posterior fossa brain malformations, hemangiomas, arterial anomalies, coarctation of the aorta and cardiac defects, and eye abnormalities) syndrome in anywhere from 20% to 31% of cases.[14,15]

PHACE syndrome is characterized by the presence of a segmental or large facial hemangioma associated with posterior fossa and cerebral vascular anomalies as well as cardiac and ocular abnormalities.[16] A consensus group meeting in 2009 defined diagnostic criteria for PHACE syndrome.[13] These infants require additional workup, including further imaging of the head, neck, and chest and dermatologic and ophthalmologic examinations.[17] Acute ischemic stroke is a known risk in these individuals given their predilection for underlying vascular anomalies and must be considered when waging optimal treatment regimens for their tumors.[18]

Clinical course of IHs varies widely but typically follows a consistent pattern of proliferation, latency, and involution. After initiation of the proliferative phase of growth, IHs have been shown to reach approximately 80% of their final size by a mean age of 3 to 6 months.[19] By 12 months, a vast majority of IHs have entered the latent phase or have already began to involute, although there are rare cases where these tumors continue to grow past 2 years of age. As the involution phase takes over, IHs drastically shrink in size and turgidity and experience color change from red to gray and often return to a more neutral skin color over the next 5 to 7 years.[20]

A majority of IHs follow the described natural history of disease without need for intervention and have mostly involuted by late childhood

Table 2		
Subclassification of infantile hemangiomas based on types and patterns of distribution		
Infantile Hemangioma		
Pattern	**Types**	
Focal	Superficial	
Multifocal	Mixed/compound	
Segmental	Deep	
Indeterminate	Reticular	
Association with Other Lesions		
PHACE association		
Posterior fossa malformations, hemangioma, arterial anomalies, cardiovascular anomalies, eye anomalies, and sternal clefting and/or supraumbilical raphe		
LUMBAR association		
Lower body hemangioma, urogenital anomalies, ulceration, myelopathy, bony deformities, anorectal malformations, arterial anomalies, and renal anomalies		

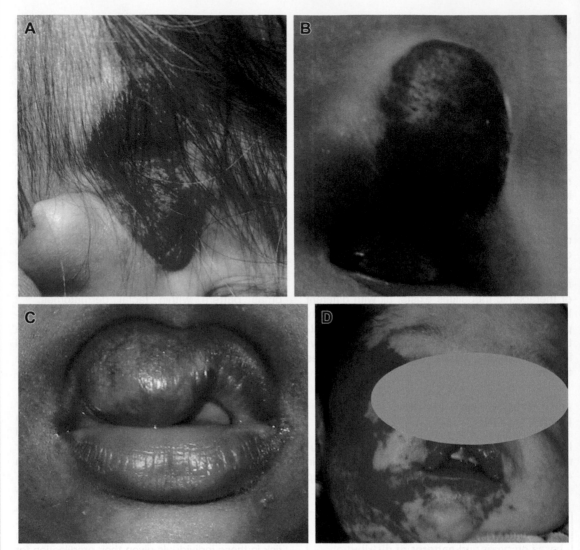

Fig. 1. Different types and patterns of distribution of IHs. (*A*) Superficial hemangioma of the postauricular skin, (*B*) compound hemangioma of the left eyebrow, (*C*) deep hemangioma of the upper lip, and (*D*) segmental hemangioma of the face warranting work-up up of PHACE diagnosis.

(approximately 50% by age 5% and 70% by age 7). Approximately 40% to 50% of children, however, are left with either residual tumor, loose and irregular skin, telangiectasias, or scarring, which may require intervention down the road for cosmesis.[21,22] It is estimated that at some point during their clinical course, approximately 10% of IHs become destructive or disfiguring or may threaten vision or airway patency; become ulcerated or infected; cause heart failure, severe thrombocytopenia, or bleeding; and, thus, be life-threatening.[23] These clinical scenarios often warrant intervention. There have been several studies that have looked at the association of clinical characteristics and predilection for developing complications to better inform need for

treatment and specialty referral—among these worrisome features are facial location, segmental morphology, and larger size (for every 10 cm^2 of increasing size, there is a 5% increase in the likelihood of developing a complication).[24]

Given the great diversity in presentation and clinical course of these lesions, no single treatment option is ideal for all cases. The overarching goal of intervention for IHs is to maximize the functional and cosmetic result while minimizing associated morbidity and complications. Ideally this treatment goal has been achieved by 3 to 5 years of age when children have developed self-image, experience new social pressures associated with school, and have become more psychologically vulnerable.[25] Evidence-based therapies for the treatment of IHs re reviewed in detail later.

WATCH AND WAIT

As discussed previously, a majority of IH patients (approximately 60%) do not require medical or surgical treatment because their lesions are self-involuting and never pose permanent cosmetic, functional, or psychological morbidity. In these cases, a conservative approach of parental reassurance, close follow-up, and routine monitoring for clinical changes is sufficient.[26] In general, it is acceptable practice to watch these lesions until intervention is predicted to lead to a better outcome than allowing a tumor to follow its natural course of disease.[27] In cases where surgical intervention might be warranted, waiting for complete involution may offer the benefit of increased skin availability, better scar location and size, and smaller risk of damage to adjacent structures.[23] With the advent of propranolol, the modern-day trend is a gravitation of parents and practitioners toward early pharmacologic intervention for a greater range of tumors than ever before, and, therefore, the watch-and-wait approach may be losing popularity.[27,28]

STEROIDS—SYSTEMIC/INTRALESIONAL

Until the first use of propranolol in 2008, both systemic and IL steroids had been a mainstay of treatment of IHs. Systemic and intralesional (IL) steroids had proved effective but not without causing substantial side effects, although mainly short term, including growth disturbances, infections, personality changes, cushingoid facies, and immunosuppression.[22,29,30] The majority of literature supporting steroid use is level IV–V evidence in the form of small case series and observational and retrospective studies. A study by Enjolras and colleagues[31] showed that steroids bring about significant tumor improvement in approximately 30% of patients, another 30% show no change and ultimately require dose increases to 5 mg/kg per day, and 40% experience partial/minimal responses (level V evidence). Pandey and colleagues[32] reviewed their institution's 20 year experience with these modalities (level IV evidence). A total of 2013 patients received either oral steroids (499 patients), IL steroids (886 patients), or a combination for these modalities (628 patients). Results revealed that superficial hemangiomas responded best to all treatment modalities—95% had greater than 75 to 50% regression versus 90% of mixed and 70% of deep lesions (P<.01 for superficial vs deep responses). Children

less than 1 year of age showed statistically significant better response than older children. The complications of treatment were local infections related to ulceration (12.4%, not statistically different between the 3 groups); cushingoid facies/growth delay and hypertension (3.1% and 2.5%, respectively, statistically more frequent in the dual-modality and systemic steroid groups). The investigators recommended that for smaller lesions ($\leq$25 cm^2), IL therapy should be first choice, regardless of hemangioma type (superficial, deep, or mixed). Oral therapy was recommended as the initial choice for larger ($\geq$25 cm^2) or multiple tumors and combined therapy for nonresponders to IL therapy.[32] Many other investigators have provided level V evidence that is in agreement with Pandey and colleagues' advocacy for the use of IL steroids for small localized hemangiomas where directed injections can cause tumor response without the systemic side effects of other pharmacotherapies.[33,34]

Recognizing the lack of higher-level evidence supporting steroid use for IHs, Bennett and colleagues[35] designed a meta-analysis in 2001 compiling data from 10 case series, including 184 patients with IHs who were treated with systemic glucocorticoids (level III evidence). The investigation found a response rate of 84% and a rebound rate of 36%. Adverse events were reported in 34% of cases independent of dosing. In the first small RCT to provide level II evidence looking at efficacy of oral steroids for IH treatment, Pope and colleagues[36] randomized 20 patients with problematic IHs to either daily oral prednisolone or monthly intravenous pulses of methylprednisolone. Improvement using a visual analog score that estimates overall changes in size and adverse events were compared at 3 months from baseline and 1 year of age. The investigators found that oral prednisone therapy resulted in improved resolution but had a higher rate of adverse events compared with pulse dosing.[36]

Highlighting the substantial difference in safety profile between corticosteroids and propranolol, Sawa and colleagues[37] performed a prospective database analysis (level IV evidence) to describe the long-term effects of steroids versus β-blockers on anthropometric measurements in 18 children with IHs. The investigators found a significant increase in body mass index and decrease in height percentile in children treated with steroids. The propranolol group required longer duration of therapy and had significantly lower systolic blood pressures but without symptomatic hypotension.[37] Additionally, Price and colleagues[38] supported propranolol's efficacy to be superior to steroids and to lead to significantly less relapses and less need for surgical intervention as well as lower cost and side effects (level IV evidence). Although substantial evidence exists supporting the efficacy of steroids for management of IHs, their poor side-effect profile is well-supported in the literature and has led to a dramatic shift in management over the past 5 years toward β-blocker therapy as the preferred treatment modality for IHs. This shift is not only obvious when reviewing the literature but also has been demonstrated to exist within individual institutions as is shown by level V evidence from Gomulka and colleagues.[39]

PROPRANOLOL

Propranolol hydrochloride, a nonselective β-blocker, is rapidly becoming the mainstay of treatment of IHs. In a landmark *New England Journal of Medicine* article from 2008, Léauté-Labrèze and colleagues[40] published a small case series inspired by patients treated with propranolol for cardiopulmonary purposes who were incidentally noted to have response of their IHs to the drug (level V evidence). Within a year of this first report by Léauté-Labrèze and colleagues, several level V reports further confirmed the efficacy of propranolol for management of airway IHs.[41–43] A subsequent series of 32 cases by Sans and colleagues[44] reported immediate effect of propranolol treatment on color and growth of IHs leading to considerable shortening of the course of disease (level V evidence). Whereas most prior studies had looked at treatment of IHs in the proliferative phase, Zvulunov and colleagues'[45] retrospective study showed that latent or involuting tumors treated with propranolol experience faster rates of involution compared with untreated tumors (level V evidence). The first larger 2010 retrospective review by Buckmiller and colleagues[46] showed that among 32 patients with IHs, 97% demonstrated response to propranolol therapy and half did not require any further treatment (level V evidence). These studies reported that therapy was overall well tolerated, with only minor side effects, such as gastrointestinal reflux disease, somnolence, respiratory syncytial virus exacerbation, and rash. Several investigators continued to report their experiences in 2010 to 2011 through mainly level V evidence, including case reports and series, all supporting the efficacy and excellent safety profile of propranolol and endorsing its use as a first-line therapy for management of these tumors (**Fig. 2**).[22,38,45,47,48] As the efficacy and safety profile of propranolol became largely supported by level IV–V evidence during the early years after its discovery in 2008, higher levels of

evidence were still needed to justify its widespread use.

After these observational and retrospective studies, several investigators recognized the need for a large meta-analysis and randomized controlled trials (RCTs) to further prove efficacy, and establish criteria for administration. Hogeling and colleagues[49] compared 24 weeks of propranolol with placebo in the treatment of 40 children ages 9 weeks to 5 years with facial or potentially disfiguring IHS (level II evidence). In this RCT, the investigators found a significant reduction in IH redness and elevations at weeks 12 and 24 of treatment in the propranolol group versus placebo ($P<.01$ and $P<.001$, respectively), with no serious adverse effects reported.[49]

A meta-analysis from 2011 compiling 213 patients from 49 articles described a common approach and course of treatment when using propranolol for management of IHs (level III evidence).[50] In this study, 93% of patients had therapy initiated in infancy at a mean age of 4.5 months. Initiation of therapy was closely monitored in all studies but with different approaches — some practiced inpatient monitoring whereas others implemented close outpatient monitoring with frequent follow-up. Dosing in 65% of patients was 2 mg/kg/d, and in 25% of patients 3 mg/kg/d, for an average duration of 5.1 months.[50] Without any clear guidelines for propranolol use at the time, this meta-analysis unveiled the discrepancies in how treating physicians were managing IHs with β-blockers and underscored the need for more uniform consensus.

There have been several more recent, well-designed meta-analyses and RCTs conducted in the past few years showing direct superiority of propranolol over steroids for IHs.[51–53] Malik and colleagues[51] designed a RCT comparing the efficacy of orally administered propranolol versus systemic steroids versus using both medications concurrently. The investigators showed that propranolol brought about earlier improved changes and that there was no significant increased benefit of adding prednisolone to propranolol, but this addition did lead to poorer patient compliance secondary to a higher number of complications associated with steroid use.[51] A meta-analysis in 2013 pooled data from 1965 to 2012, resulting in a comparison of 2697 patients from 16 studies who had received oral or locally administered glucocorticoids with 795 pooled patients from 25 studies who had been treated with propranolol (level II evidence).[53] Systemic glucocorticoids had an overall efficacy of 71% versus 97% for treatment with propranolol. Furthermore, the study revealed that steroid complication rate was double

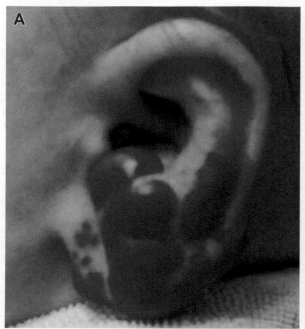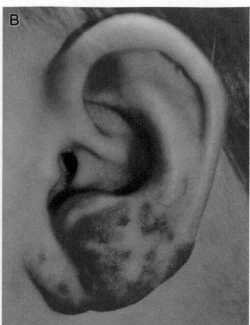

Fig. 2. Example of a left ear IH treated with propranolol. (*A*) Left ear appearance at 3 months of age prior to propranolol treatment. (*B*) Left ear appearance after 3 months of propranolol treatment.

that of propranolol therapy (23% vs 9.6%, respectively).[53] Most recently, a 2014 phase 2, investigator-blinded, multi-institutional RCT was published comparing propranolol and prednisolone in the management of IHs. The study was terminated prior to targeted enrollment secondary to adverse events, leading to withdrawal in the prednisolone-treated group (level II evidence).[52]

Overall, there exists substantial level IV–V evidence in the form of observational and retrospective studies as well as some level II–III evidence in the form of meta-analyses and RCTs, providing physicians with adequate evidence-based support for the efficacy and safety of propranolol as a first-line treatment of IHs. In return, the Food and Drug Administration (FDA) has recently approved Hemangeol, (Pierre Fabre Pharmaceuticals, Inc, Parsippany, NJ, USA) a liquid suspension of propranolol, as the first-ever FDA approved treatment option for proliferating IHs. This approval was based largely on double-blinded RCT.[54] In this phase II/III trial, 460 infants were randomized to receive placebo or 1 of 4 dosing regimens (1.2 or 3.4 mg/kg/d in twice-daily divided doses for 3 or for 6 months) of Hemangeol.[54] At 24 weeks, treatment response was evaluated by blinded, centralized, independent assessments of photographs compared with baseline. The trial showed that 60% of infants treated with Hemangeol versus 4% of those treated with placebo, met the primary endpoint of complete or near-complete resolution of the IH (*P* = .0001).

The most frequently reported adverse reactions in the treatment group were sleep disorders (16.1% vs 5.9% in placebo) and aggravated respiratory tract infections, such as bronchitis and bronchiolitis (13% vs 4.7% in placebo), leading to treatment discontinuation in fewer than 2% of patients. Current absolute contraindications for the use of Hemangeol are prematurity (corrected age <5 weeks), infants weighing less than 2 kg, known hypersensitivity to propranolol, asthma or history of bronchospasm, heart rate less than 80 beats per minute, decompensated heart failure, greater than first-degree heart block, blood pressure less than 50/30 mm Hg, and pheochromocytoma (**Box 1**). A barrier to its widespread clinical use is its exceedingly high cost, which raises the question of whether Hemangeol has any increased efficacy over generic liquid propranolol and other β-blocker alternatives. In a recent, small RCT, 23 IH patients were randomized to receive either propranolol or atenolol and a noninferiority analysis was conducted. When comparing complete responses (60% in propranolol group and 53.8% in the atenolol group; *P* = .68) and side-effect profiles of these 2 β-blockers in the treatment of IHs, there were no significant differences.[55]

Considering the great variability in propranolol treatment protocols used by physicians, Drolet and colleagues[11] arranged a 2013 consensus conference to discuss evidence-based recommendations for propranolol dosing administration and safety/toxicity monitoring. Key dosing regimens from this consensus statement are highlighted in **Fig. 3**. Regarding when to treat IHs with propranolol, the investigators recommended individualized decision making based on lesion characteristics and predicted disease course but encouraged intervention in cases of ulceration; of impairment of vital functions, such as ocular or airway involvement; and when permanent disfigurement is considered a possibility. When planning initiation of β-blocker therapy, they recommended pretreatment risk screening, including recent cardiovascular and pulmonary screen as well as blood pressure and heart rate assessment. Use of pretreatment ECG in all infants with IHs did not achieve consensus but was recommended as part of the cardiovascular work-up in cases of low heart rate for age or presence of an auscultated arrhythmia, family history of congenital heart defects or arrhythmias, and maternal history of a connective tissue disorder (see **Box 1**). In terms of propranolol use in patients with PHACE syndrome, these patients are often ideal candidates for propranolol therapy given their large facial hemangiomas and predilection for scarring, but their coexisting medical complexities and risk for acute ischemic events raises controversy

A

Inpatient Initiation of Propranolol: Suggested for infants <8 weeks of gestationally corrected age or with comorbid conditions

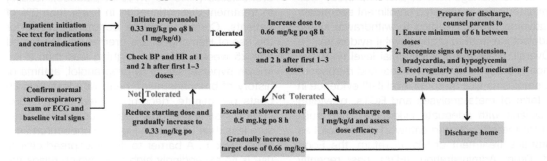

B

Outpatient Initiation of Propranolol: Suggested for infants >8 weeks of gestationally corrected age and adequate social support

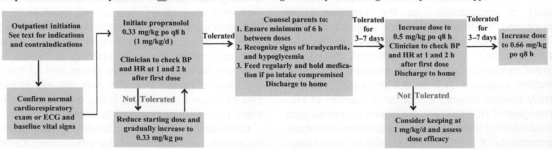

Fig. 3. Summary of recommended dosing for (*A*) inpatient and (*B*) outpatient initiation of propranolol for IHs. BP, blood pressure; HR, heart rate. (*Adapted from* Drolet BA, Frommelt PC, Chamlin SL, et al. Initiation and use of propranolol for infantile hemangioma: report of a consensus conference. Pediatrics 2013;131(1):135; with permission.)

over its use. The consensus group encouraged MRI/echocardiography/other vascular imaging in any patients who may be at risk for PHACE syndrome, and in any patient found to have underlying vascular anomalies, consultation with cardiology and neurology should be obtained for comanagement during treatment. Propranolol should be initiated when benefits are thought to outweigh risks in PHACE syndrome patients, and the consensus group advocates for use of lowest-possible dosing, slow up-titration of doses, 3 times daily dosing to minimize blood pressure effects, and inpatient monitoring of high-risk individuals.

Target dosing, of 2 mg/kg/d divided in 3 daily doses, 6 hours apart, should be achieved after a slow dose escalation in all patients. Those infants who are less than 8 weeks of gestationally corrected age, who have poor social support, or who have any cardiovascular or pulmonary comorbid conditions should have their dosing initiated as inpatients for closer monitoring (see **Fig. 3**). The outpatient setting is appropriate for infants who do not meet these criteria. Outpatient monitoring includes heart rate and blood pressure checks 1 and 2 hours after each new dose escalation and extensive counseling of parents regarding home administration of the medication and worrisome signs/symptoms to look out for. Neither routine use of Holter monitoring nor evaluation for asymptomatic hypoglycemia was recommended by the consensus group given poor evidence-based support for these interventions. Lastly, the group advocates for discontinuation of propranolol during times of concurrent illness to prevent hypoglycemia when oral intake may be poor. The consensus group made conservative evidence-based recommendations about preoperative evaluation, dosing regimens, initiation, and monitoring, although stressed that given the persistent lack of evidence in certain areas, much of their consensus was still based on expert opinion and experience.[11]

TOPICAL/INTRALESIONAL β-BLOCKERS

Topical β-blocker regimens have recently been investigated as an alternative to systemic therapy in children with small superficial IHs or with contraindications to systemic propranolol. Patients who experience adverse side effects from oral therapy, which may include hypotension and bradycardia; respiratory issues, such as bronchospasm and wheezing; sleep disturbances (related to propranolol's ability to cross the blood-brain barrier); and diarrhea, are also potential candidates for trials of topical therapy. Prior research has shown systemic absorption of topical β-blockers to be

minimal to nonexistent, thus affording them an excellent safety profile associated with limited side effects.[56,57] Current evidence for topical β-blocker treatment of IHs includes a host of small retrospective, observational, prospective cohort studies (level IV–V evidence), 2 RCTs (level II evidence), and a recent meta-analysis (level II evidence). Xu and colleagues[58] showed 90% either good or partial responses and 10% were nonresponders to topical 1% propranolol in their level V review of 28 superficial IHs. No systemic side effects were seen. In an RCT randomizing 5- to 24-week-olds with superficial, nonulcerated IHs to either placebo or treatment with topical 0.5% timolol, the treatment group had a significantly greater reduction in size and volume of the tumors than the untreated group.[59] Another 2013 RCT randomized 45 patients with IHs to receive oral propranolol, topical 1% propranolol ointment, or IL propranolol (15 patients in each group), and assessed outcomes at 6 months once all treatments had ended.[60] The oral propranolol group had excellent responses in 60% of patients, whereas the topical ointment and intralesional groups demonstrated excellent responses in only 20% and 13.3%, respectively ($P = .04$). No adverse side effects were encountered other than pain/inconvenience of therapy associated with IL therapy, causing 3 of those patients to drop out.[60]

By 2014, various case series and small retrospective/prospective reviews exploring topical therapy for IHs had been published reporting a range of outcomes. These led to a 2015 meta-analysis that reviewed 94 articles pertaining to topical β-blockers for treatment of superficial IHs.[57] A total of 17 of these were reports describing management of 5 or more patients treated with topical application of timolol, topical propranolol, or IL injection of propranolol for superficial, cutaneous IHs. Data from a total of 554 patients from all studies were pooled for analysis. Response rates (defined as a clinically significant response) for topical propranolol and topical timolol were not significantly different, 76% versus 83%, respectively ($P = .45$). The investigators were unable to calculate a meta-effects estimate of IL therapy secondary to overall lack of available evidence and significant variability in reported effects.[57] This meta-analysis represent strong level II evidence supporting good clinical efficacy and excellent safety profile of topical β-blockers in the treatment of superficial IHs. On the other hand, use of topical therapy for the treatment of deep or compound IHs has not been shown similarly efficacious.[61–63]

Although the average response rates of approximately 70% to 80% for topical therapies in the treatment of superficial IHs approach but do not exceed those of oral propranolol (approximately 88%–97%[53,54]), their safety profile is superior, and, therefore, they should be considered a reasonable option in patients with contraindications to or poor tolerance of oral therapy. Some investigators have suggested topical propranolol/timolol as first-line treatment of superficial lesions and, in cases of poor response, subsequently switching to oral agents.[57] Currently, there is strong level I–II evidence supporting the efficacy and safety profile of topical β-blocker therapy for the treatment of superficial IHs. Further studies are needed to investigate superiority of different dosing regimens, use of higher pharmacologic concentrations that could presumably improve efficacy for deep or compound lesions without effecting safety, and potential benefit of combination oral and topical β-blocker therapy.

SURGERY

For the approximately 40% of patients who require intervention for their IHs,[24] surgery is reserved for a subset of these based on certain clinical features of their disease. Patients who experience IH-related complications, have functionally impairing lesions, or fail medical therapy may ultimately require surgery (**Fig. 4**). Evidence directly comparing outcomes of surgical intervention with other modalities is lacking. To date, there is scant level IV–V evidence, including a few retrospective reviews,[64–66] that focuses on indications and outcomes of surgical intervention without any well-powered RCTs or meta-analyses. In a 2005 report from a national research workshop for IHs, indications for surgical intervention were delineated based on tumor phase.[67] The consortium recommended that tumors in the proliferating phase should undergo surgery when they cause airway or visual obstruction, craniofacial deformation, recurrent bleeding, or ulceration unresponsive to medical therapy. Indications for surgical excision of tumors in the involution and involuted phases are (1) when resection or reconstruction are

considered inevitable or (2) for excision of contour deformities involving damaged skin or fibrofatty residuum (**Fig. 5**).[67] Although these recommended indications provide some guidance about the clinical scenarios when surgery is clearly necessary, treating physicians still struggle with timing of surgery and with how to predict which tumors require surgery. In a retrospective study looking at ideal timing for resection of 21 lip IHs, Hynes and colleagues[64] showed that early operative intervention during the proliferative phase (rather than waiting for involution) resulted in better outcomes. Those patients who were operated on earlier had significantly fewer IH-related complications, including less bleeding, ulceration, and speech impairment, and fewer feeding difficulties and psychosocial issues. These investigators, among others, advocate for earlier intervention to avoid later development of such complications.[68,69] Predictability of future need for surgical intervention based on aspects of disease course and characteristics has only recently been studied.[66] Lee and colleagues[66] recognized the potential benefit of identifying early characteristics of IHs that could serve to inform physicians about the likelihood of needing future resection. In their retrospective review of 112 IHs undergoing surgery, the investigators found that females, premature infants, and tumors of the head and neck (vs below the neck) were significantly more likely to undergo surgery. Overall, decision for surgical intervention in cases of IHs is largely based on the individual clinical experience of the treating surgeon and is weakly supported by a handful of retrospective reviews and case reports in the literature.

PULSED DYE LASER THERAPY

Various laser therapy options exist for the treatment of IHs, with varying degrees of evidence supporting their efficacy. The pulsed dye laser (PDL) is currently the most popular laser used in treating IHs of the head and neck. In a process called selective photothermolysis,[70] it works through

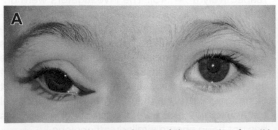 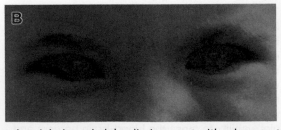

Fig. 4. Functionally impairing IH. (*A*) Example of an IH causing right lateral globe displacement with subsequent vision impairment. Patient was minimally responsive to delayed initiation of propranolol therapy and required surgical intervention. (*B*) Postoperative photograph of right eye after surgical resection of hemangioma resulting in correction of globe position and vision.

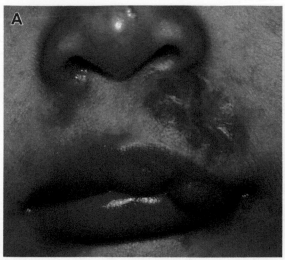
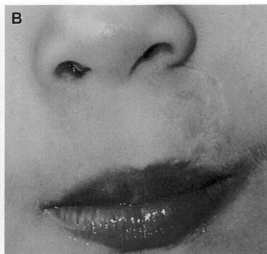

Fig. 5. Involuted IH. (*A*) Photograph of an upper lip IH after undergoing involution. The quality of the residual skin is loose, irregular, and cosmetically deforming, thus warranting surgical intervention. (*B*) Postoperative results of the involuted upper lip hemangioma after tissue resection and advancement, resulting in an improved cosmetic appearance.

emission of short pulses of light, at a wavelength of 585 to 595 nm, that are absorbed by oxyhemoglobin, resulting in thermal destruction of vascular lesions but sparing normal surrounding tissue. The PDL is capable of a 1.2-mm depth of penetration and is, therefore, reserved mainly for superficial hemangiomas. Clinically it is used to reduce redness of proliferating lesions and to potentially limit overall growth size.[27] Complications of IHs, such as ulceration and pain, have also been treated with PDLs, with only uncontrolled, retrospective or small prospective evidence supporting its use for these purposes.[71–74] PDLs are generally well tolerated—side effects of their use for treatment of IHs include temporary local swelling, hyper- or hypopigmentation, and rarely pain, scarring, ulceration, or hemorrhage.[75]

The PDL has been used and studied for more than 30 years as an option for treatment of IHs, and, as a result, there is substantial level III–V evidence in the form of various case reports, retrospective reviews, and small, nonrandomized prospective studies supporting its efficacy in the literature.[76–83] In 2002, the first level III evidence comparing PDL therapy to observation in the treatment of IHs was performed by Batta and colleagues[84] and raised significant doubt surrounding its efficacy. The investigators' analysis revealed no benefit in the number of children whose lesions showed complete clearance or minimal residual signs at 1 year in the PDL versus observation group. Furthermore, the PDL-treated lesions experienced significantly more skin atrophy and hypopigmentation. As a result of these

findings, use of the PDL for treatment of IHs remains controversial, although more modern cooling techniques and use of larger spot sizes are now available, a fact that some believe render Batta and colleagues' findings obsolete.

More recent integrated cooling techniques have brought about PDLs that use higher and more effective energy output regimens that also achieve deeper tissue penetration. Two studies, a level II prospective RCT[80] and a level V retrospective review,[81] have shown increased efficacy in the treatment of IHs with these lasers. Despite the availability of newer, more effective lasers, the literature still supports the use of these instruments mainly for the treatment of superficial rather than deep IHs. In their level III, prospective, non-RCT looking at 224 hemangiomas, Poetke and colleagues[79] showed that superficial hemangiomas responded best to PDL treatment (86% had excellent or good results) and that deep components of mixed hemangiomas did not respond in any cases. A complicating factor in the interpretation of the current evidence for PDL treatment of IHs is that the studies that do show similar outcomes often use discrepant laser settings and therapy regimens, making them difficult to compare.[75] Furthermore, many of the lasers have experienced drastic changes over time based on technological advances, and, therefore, older studies using older technology may no longer be clinically relevant. More recent studies, using cooling technologies and larger spot sizes, are showing promise in the management of superficial hemangiomas.

Table 3
Evidence for alternative treatment modalities for infantile hemangiomas

Modality	Author (Year)	Level of Evidence, Study Design	N	Findings
Systemic				
Interferon-alpha (IFN)	Michaud et al,[95] 2004	Level II, metanalysis	3113 Children <18 y old treated with IFN for chronic hepatitis (69%) or vascular tumors (14%)	IFN should not be used in infants under 1 y of age unless for life-threatening tumors unresponsive to other treatments. When IFN is used, children should have monthly neurologic examinations.
	Dubois et al,[94] 1999	Level III, prospective cohort	53 Infants with severe hemangiomas	Toxicity was generally mild and transient grade 1 toxicity occurred in 100%, grade 2 toxicity in 89%, grade 3 toxicity in 58%, and grade 4 toxicity in 17%. Severe neurotoxicity in the form of spastic diplegia occurred in 1 patient.
	Barlow et al,[93] 1998	Level IV, case series	Of 26 patients treated with interferon, 5 infants who developed spastic diplegia were selected.	IFN can adversely affect the immature central nervous system and produce spastic diplegia—potentially reversible. Recommended careful clinical assessment of neurodevelopmental status during IFN therapy.
	Tamayo et al,[91] 1997	Level IV, case series	7 Infants with organ-interfering/life-threatening giant hemangiomas	Considerable reduction of the volume of the hemangiomas and remission of IH complications. Side effects of fever, neutropenia, and an increase in serum aminotransferase levels were seen.
	Ezekowitz et al,[92] 1992	Level IV, case series	20 Neonates and infants with life-threatening or vision-threatening hemangiomas that failed to respond to corticosteroid therapy	18 Of the 20 hemangiomas, regressed by 50% or more after an average of 7.8 mo of treatment. Side effects included fever, neutropenia (1 patient), and skin necrosis (1 patient).

Vincristine	Enjolras et al,[96] 2004	Level IV, case series	9 Infants with life-endangering hemangiomas	7 Patients had a clear clinical response at end of first month of treatment, whereas other 2 demonstrated slower response. Transient mild side effects were present in 4 patients.
	Fawcett et al,[98] 2004	Level IV, case report	1 Large, steroid-resistant IH of head and neck	Significant clinical improvement with therapy.
	Perez et al,[97] 2002	Level IV, case series	3 Children with life-endangering hemangiomas refractory to steroids	Suggest that vincristine is an effective alternative in the treatment of corticosteroid-resistant, life-threatening IHs. During treatment and follow-up, did not observe any toxicity related to vincristine treatment.
	Moore et al,[99] 2001	Level IV, case report	1 Airway hemangioma, refractory to steroids	Dramatic improvement with vincristine.
Cyclophosphamide	Fukushima et al,[100] 2011	Level IV, case report	1 Patient with life-threatening hepatic hemangioma and multiple cutaneous hemangiomas	Successfully treated with corticosteroid, interferon-alpha, embolization, and cyclophosphamide. Suggest cyclophosphamide in a multimodal approach may be effective.
	Gottschling et al,[102] 2006	Level IV, case series	2 Patients with life-threatening IH	Improvement of both infants.
	Sovinz et al,[103] 2006	Level IV, case report	1 Infant with IH	Successfully treated with corticosteroid, interferon-alpha, hepatic embolization, and cyclophosphamide.
	Hurvitz et al,[101] 2000	Level IV, case report	1 Infant with life-threatening diffuse hemangiomatosis of liver, refractory to steroids	Successful treatment of tumor burden, no long-term adverse effects.

(continued on next page)

Table 3
(continued)

Modality	Author (Year)	Level of Evidence, Study Design	N	Findings
Topical				
Imiquimod	Qiu et al,[105] 2013	Level IV, retrospective review	20 Superficial IHs treated with timolol vs 20 superficial IHs treated with imiquimod	Both imiquimod 5% cream and timolol 0.5% ophthalmic solution showed equivalent clinical efficacy after 4 mo of treatment. Timolol seemed to have fewer AEs (crusting, superficial scars, skin pigmentation) than imiquimod in the management of superficial IHs.
	Jiang et al,[107] 2011	Level II, self-controlled, prospective phase II study	44 Uncomplicated, proliferative superficial or mixed IHs (half of lesions were treated with topical agent, other half left untreated)	Effective rate was 80% (n = 35). Overall resolution rated as excellent or good rate in 39% of lesions. Relapse rate was 2%. Side effects were noted in 61% edema, local itching, peeling, erosion, crusting, ulceration, and scarring.
	Barry et al,[108] 2008	Level IV, case series	5 IHs	Good efficacy, limited side effects (skin pigmentation and scarring).
	Hazen et al,[106] 2005	Level IV, case report	1 Case of a proliferating IH	Complete resolution of lesion after 10 wk and was well tolerated.
	Martinez et al,[104] 2002	Level IV, case series	2 Cases of IHs	Resolution within 3–5 mo of therapy, minimal to no adverse effects.

Laser				
1064-nm Nd:YAG	Burns et al,[109] 2009	Level IV–V, case report, expert opinion	2 Patients treated with IHs treated with Nd:YAG, expert experience	Nd:YAG treatment can be extremely valuable in decreasing the bulk of IHs once in the involution phase (avoid in proliferative phase secondary to ulceration and skin necrosis). Its deeper penetration is effective on deep components of IHs. Morbidity, such as blistering, nonspecific tissue heating, and scarring, is much more of a possibility than with the cooled PDL.
	Ulrich et al,[110] 2005	Level IV, retrospective review	15 Patients with hemangiomas and 5 patients with vascular malformations	In the hemangioma group, 3 cases showed near-complete remission (>90%), 10 cases had a partial reduction in size (50%–90%), in 1 case there was stable disease, and in 1 case tumor growth. Adverse effects included scars (40%), hyper- and hypopigmentation (23%), mild atrophy (20%), and wrinkled texture (17%). 30% Of patients were unsatisfied and went on to surgical excision.
	Clymer et al,[111] 1998	Level III, prospective, nonrandomized cohort	10 Patients with hemangioma or vascular malformation being cotreated with systemic or intralesional steroids	Long-term follow-up showed regression of the lesion in all 10 patients with good cosmetic outcomes. The range of reduction in size was 20%–98%. No re-expansion of the lesions was noted after a mean follow-up of 13 mo.

MULTIMODALITY

Multimodality, combination therapy is a popular approach for the treatment of IHs. Combining systemic pharmacologic regimens of propranolol, steroids, or other topical alternatives with either surgery or laser treatments is common practice to optimize treatment of different lesion components. For example, physicians often treat compound hemangiomas with propranolol (which addresses the deep component) and PDL for treatment of any superficial skin involvement.[27] There are a multitude of studies looking at different modality combinations for optimal treatment of IHs, but again most of these encompass no more than level IV–V evidence.[85–89] With the advent of propranolol, more recent studies look at combinations of propranolol with topical agents, surgery, or lasers. In a level V, retrospective review of facial-segmental IHs, blinded physicians observed that those lesions treated with combination therapy (propranolol and PDL) achieved complete clearance more often (P = .01) and achieved near-complete clearance faster (P<.001) than those treated with propranolol alone.[86] In a small RCT, Ehsani and colleagues[90] randomized 19 patients to receive either PDL alone or PDL with propranolol (level II evidence). The therapeutic efficacies of each regimen were judged to have undergone either excellent, good, weak, or no clearance through a comparison of photographs of skin lesions before and after the treatment. The investigators found that 50% of dual-modality–treated patients experienced excellent clearance versus 22% in the PDL-alone group.[90] These studies collectively support a multimodal approach over any single therapy alone for the treatment of IHs because they can achieve greater efficacy and fewer side effects by reducing the individual doses of each modality necessary to bring about clinically significant responses. Larger RCTs and meta-analyses are currently lacking that would allow for grade A recommendations regarding the use of multiple modalities for the treatment of IHs.

SUMMARY

Clinicians and researchers have entered an age of medicine where the expectation is that treatment decisions and algorithms are based on high-quality evidence. Although in an ideal world, large, blinded RCTs and systematic reviews would be available that provide clear answers to clinical questions, more often than not, this is not the reality. When asking how best to treat IHs, an inundation of the literature is found, with more than 2000 studies spanning 50 years, most of which are small case series and retrospective reviews that provide weak, level III–V evidence. For example, in 2014 alone, there were more than 70 studies listed in PubMed pertaining to propranolol treatment of IHs—this equates to a new study published approximately every 5 days for the entire year. Fortunately, over the past few years, a few large RCTs and meta-analyses have arrived, which have provided higher levels of evidence, and ultimately led to the first-ever FDA approval of a treatment of IHs. Although Hemangeol™ and its oral β-blocker counterparts have solidified their role as first-line agents in the treatment of IHs, new level II evidence is showing promise for topical β-blocker agents and PDL lasers as effective alternative or adjunctive therapies with superior safety profiles. In cases of known contraindications to, or intolerance of, β-blockers, both systemic and IL steroids remain a reasonable choice. Surgical intervention is reserved for specific indications and, at this point, is largely up to the discretion of the treating physician. Other therapies, not discussed in detail, such as interferon-α,[91–95] vincristine,[96–99] cyclophosphamide,[100–103] topical imiquimod,[104–108] and the 1064-nm Nd:YAG laser,[109–111] among others, are currently reserved for life-threatening lesions or those unresponsive to conventional therapy (Table 3). These therapies are mainly supported by case series and small reviews, and, until physicians see higher levels of evidence proving their efficacy and safety profiles, it will remain unclear whether or not they could serve additional roles in the treatment of IHs. To date, there is not yet level I evidence in the form of a large, systematic review of RCTs that addresses treatment of IHs—surely this will come as more well-conducted RCTs are performed in the future. More than likely, what will be seen with these studies is that multimodality algorithms, specifically addressing individual components of these tumors, will result in the best functional and cosmetic outcomes. Treating physicians are obligated to remain privy to current evidence-based recommendations for management of IHs while using their own clinical judgment and experience in optimizing their treatment of IHs.

ACKNOWLEDGMENTS

We would like to thank Jonathan Isley for his help with figure formatting for this article.

REFERENCES

1. Mulliken JB, Glowacki J. Hemangiomas and vascular malformations in infants and children: a

classification based on endothelial characteristics. Plast Reconstr Surg 1982;69(3):412–22.

2. ISSVA.2014. Available at: issva.org/classification. Accessed January 26, 2015.

3. Leon-Villapalos J, Wolfe K, Kangesu L. GLUT-1: an extra diagnostic tool to differentiate between haemangiomas and vascular malformations. Br J Plast Surg 2005;58(3):348–52.

4. North PE, Waner M, Mizeracki A, et al. GLUT1: a newly discovered immunohistochemical marker for juvenile hemangiomas. Hum Pathol 2000;31(1):11–22.

5. Kanada KN, Merin MR, Munden A, et al. A prospective study of cutaneous findings in newborns in the United States: correlation with race, ethnicity, and gestational status using updated classification and nomenclature. J Pediatr 2012; 161(2):240–5.

6. Jacobs AH. Strawberry hemangiomas; the natural history of the untreated lesion. Calif Med 1957;86(1):8–10.

7. Enjolras O, Gelbert F. Superficial hemangiomas: associations and management. Pediatr Dermatol 1997;14(3):173–9.

8. Drolet BA, Esterly NB, Frieden IJ. Hemangiomas in children. N Engl J Med 1999;341(3):173–81.

9. Finn MC, Glowacki J, Mulliken JB. Congenital vascular lesions: clinical application of a new classification. J Pediatr Surg 1983;18(6):894–900.

10. Liang MG, Frieden IJ. Infantile and congenital hemangiomas. Semin Pediatr Surg 2014;23(4):162–7.

11. Drolet BA, Frommelt PC, Chamlin SL, et al. Initiation and use of propranolol for infantile hemangioma: report of a consensus conference. Pediatrics 2013;131(1):128–40.

12. Haggstrom AN, Lammer EJ, Schneider RA, et al. Patterns of infantile hemangiomas: new clues to hemangioma pathogenesis and embryonic facial development. Pediatrics 2006;117(3):698–703.

13. Metry D, Heyer G, Hess C, et al. Consensus statement on diagnostic criteria for PHACE syndrome. Pediatrics 2009;124(5):1447–56.

14. Metry DW, Haggstrom AN, Drolet BA, et al. A prospective study of PHACE syndrome in infantile hemangiomas: demographic features, clinical findings, and complications. Am J Med Genet A 2006;140(9):975–86.

15. Haggstrom AN, Garzon MC, Baselga E, et al. Risk for PHACE syndrome in infants with large facial hemangiomas. Pediatrics 2010;126(2):e418–26.

16. Frieden IJ, Reese V, Cohen D. PHACE syndrome. The association of posterior fossa brain malformations, hemangiomas, arterial anomalies, coarctation of the aorta and cardiac defects, and eye abnormalities. Arch Dermatol 1996;132(3): 307–11.

17. Metry DW, Dowd CF, Barkovich AJ, et al. The many faces of PHACE syndrome. J Pediatr 2001;139(1): 117–23.

18. Siegel DH, Tefft KA, Kelly T, et al. Stroke in children with posterior fossa brain malformations, hemangiomas, arterial anomalies, coarctation of the aorta and cardiac defects, and eye abnormalities (PHACE) syndrome: a systematic review of the literature. Stroke 2012;43(6):1672–4.

19. Chang LC, Haggstrom AN, Drolet BA, et al. Growth characteristics of infantile hemangiomas: implications for management. Pediatrics 2008;122(2): 360–7.

20. Boon LM, Enjolras O, Mulliken JB. Congenital hemangioma: evidence of accelerated involution. J Pediatr 1996;128(3):329–35.

21. Gampper TJ, Morgan RF. Vascular anomalies: hemangiomas. Plast Reconstr Surg 2002;110(2): 572–85 [quiz: 586]; [discussion: 587–8].

22. Zimmermann AP, Wiegand S, Werner JA, et al. Propranolol therapy for infantile haemangiomas: review of the literature. Int J Pediatr Otorhinolaryngol 2010; 74(4):338–42.

23. Burns AJ, Navarro JA, Cooner RD. Classification of vascular anomalies and the comprehensive treatment of hemangiomas. Plast Reconstr Surg 2009; 124(1 Suppl):69e–81e.

24. Haggstrom AN, Drolet BA, Baselga E, et al. Prospective study of infantile hemangiomas: clinical characteristics predicting complications and treatment. Pediatrics 2006;118(3):882–7.

25. Hochman M, Adams DM, Reeves TD. Current knowledge and management of vascular anomalies: I. hemangiomas. Arch Facial Plast Surg 2011;13(3): 145–51.

26. Tanner JL, Dechert MP, Frieden IJ. Growing up with a facial hemangioma: parent and child coping and adaptation. Pediatrics 1998;101(3 Pt 1):446–52.

27. Hochman M. Infantile hemangiomas: current management. Facial Plast Surg Clin North Am 2014; 22(4):509–21.

28. Püttgen KB. Diagnosis and management of infantile hemangiomas. Pediatr Clin North Am 2014; 61(2):383–402.

29. Boon LM, MacDonald DM, Mulliken JB. Complications of systemic corticosteroid therapy for problematic hemangioma. Plast Reconstr Surg 1999; 104(6):1616–23.

30. Kelly ME, Juern AM, Grossman WJ, et al. Immunosuppressive effects in infants treated with corticosteroids for infantile hemangiomas. Arch Dermatol 2010;146(7):767–74.

31. Enjolras O, Riche MC, Merland JJ, et al. Management of alarming hemangiomas in infancy: a review of 25 cases. Pediatrics 1990;85(4): 491–8.

32. Pandey A, Gangopadhyay AN, Gopal SC, et al. Twenty years' experience of steroids in infantile hemangioma–a developing country's perspective. J Pediatr Surg 2009;44(4):688–94.

33. Chen MT, Yeong EK, Horng SY. Intralesional corticosteroid therapy in proliferating head and neck
hemangiomas: a review of 155 cases. J Pediatr
Surg 2000;35(3):420–3.

34. Couto JA, Greene AK. Management of problematic
infantile hemangioma using intralesional triamcino-
lone: efficacy and safety in 100 infants. J Plast Reconstr Aesthet Surg 2014;67:1469–74.

35. Bennett ML, Fleischer AB, Chamlin SL, et al. Oral
corticosteroid use is effective for cutaneous hemangiomas: an evidence-based evaluation. Arch
Dermatol 2001;137(9):1208–13.

36. Pope E, Krafchik BR, Macarthur C, et al. Oral versus
high-dose pulse corticosteroids for problematic infantile hemangiomas: a randomized, controlled trial.
Pediatrics 2007;119(6):e1239–1247.

37. Sawa K, Yazdani A, Rieder MJ, et al. Propranolol
therapy for infantile hemangioma is less toxic but
longer in duration than corticosteroid therapy.
Can J Plast Surg 2014;22(4):233–6.

38. Price CJ, Lattouf C, Baum B, et al. Propranolol vs
corticosteroids for infantile hemangiomas: a multicenter retrospective analysis. Arch Dermatol
2011;147(12):1371–6.

39. Gomulka J, Siegel DH, Drolet BA. Dramatic shift in the
infantile hemangioma treatment paradigm at a single
institution. Pediatr Dermatol 2013;30(6):751–2.

40. Léauté-Labrèze C, Dumas de la Roque E, Hubiche T,
et al. Propranolol for severe hemangiomas of infancy.
N Engl J Med 2008;358(24):2649–51.

41. Truong MT, Chang KW, Berk DR, et al. Propranolol
for the treatment of a life-threatening subglottic and
mediastinal infantile hemangioma. J Pediatr 2010;
156(2):335–8.

42. Buckmiller L, Dyamenahalli U, Richter GT. Propranolol for airway hemangiomas: case report of
novel treatment. Laryngoscope 2009;119(10):
2051–4.

43. Denoyelle F, Leboulanger N, Enjolras O, et al. Role
of propranolol in the therapeutic strategy of infantile
laryngotracheal hemangioma. Int J Pediatr Otorhinolaryngol 2009;73(8):1168–72.

44. Sans V, de la Roque ED, Berge J, et al. Propranolol
for severe infantile hemangiomas: follow-up report.
Pediatrics 2009;124(3):e423–431.

45. Zvulunov A, McCuaig C, Frieden IJ, et al. Oral propranolol therapy for infantile hemangiomas beyond
the proliferation phase: a multicenter retrospective
study. Pediatr Dermatol 2011;28(2):94–8.

46. Buckmiller LM, Munson PD, Dyamenahalli U, et al.
Propranolol for infantile hemangiomas: early expe-
rience at a tertiary vascular anomalies center.
Laryngoscope 2010;120(4):676–81.

47. Schupp CJ, Kleber JB, Günther P, et al. Propranolol
therapy in 55 infants with infantile hemangioma:
dosage, duration, adverse effects, and outcome.
Pediatr Dermatol 2011;28(6):640–4.

48. Luo Y, Zeng Y, Zhou B, et al. A retrospective
study of propranolol therapy in 635 infants with
infantile hemangioma. Pediatr Dermatol 2014;32:
151–2.

49. Hogeling M, Adams S, Wargon O. A randomized
controlled trial of propranolol for infantile hemangiomas. Pediatrics 2011;128(2):e259–266.

50. Menezes MD, McCarter R, Greene EA, et al. Status
of propranolol for treatment of infantile hemangioma and description of a randomized clinical trial.
Ann Otol Rhinol Laryngol 2011;120(10):686–95.

51. Malik MA, Menon P, Rao KL, et al. Effect of propranolol vs prednisolone vs propranolol with prednisolone in the management of infantile hemangioma: a
randomized controlled study. J Pediatr Surg 2013;
48(12):2453–9.

52. Bauman NM, McCarter RJ, Guzzetta PC, et al. Propranolol vs prednisolone for symptomatic proliferating infantile hemangiomas: a randomized
clinical trial. JAMA Otolaryngol Head Neck Surg
2014;140(4):323–30.

53. Izadpanah A, Izadpanah A, Kanevsky J, et al. Propranolol versus corticosteroids in the treatment of
infantile hemangioma: a systematic review and
meta-analysis. Plast Reconstr Surg 2013;131(3):
601–13.

54. Léauté-Labrèze C, Hoeger P, Mazereeuw-
Hautier J, et al. A randomized, controlled trial of
oral propranolol in infantile hemangioma. N Engl J
Med 2015;372(8):735–46.

55. Ábarzúa-Araya A, Navarrete-Dechent CP,
Heusser F, et al. Atenolol versus propranolol for the
treatment of infantile hemangiomas: a randomized
controlled study. J Am Acad Dermatol 2014;70(6):
1045–9.

56. Ademola JI, Chow CA, Wester RC, et al. Metabolism of propranolol during percutaneous absorption in human skin. J Pharm Sci 1993;82(8):767–70.

57. Ovadia SA, Landy DC, Cohen ER, et al. Local
administration of β-blockers for infantile hemangiomas: a systematic review and meta-analysis.
Ann Plast Surg 2015;74(2):256–62.

58. Xu G, Lv R, Zhao Z, et al. Topical propranolol for
treatment of superficial infantile hemangiomas.
J Am Acad Dermatol 2012;67(6):1210–3.

59. Chan H, McKay C, Adams S, et al. RCT of timolol
maleate gel for superficial infantile hemangiomas
in 5- to 24-week-olds. Pediatrics 2013;131(6):
e1739–1747.

60. Zaher H, Rasheed H, Esmat S, et al. Propranolol
and infantile hemangiomas: different routes of
administration, a randomized clinical trial. Eur J
Dermatol 2013;23(5):646–52.

61. Wang L, Xia Y, Zhai Y, et al. Topical propranolol hydrochloride gel for superficial infantile hemangiomas. J Huazhong Univ Sci Technolog Med Sci
2012;32(6):923–6.

62. Chakkittakandiyil A, Phillips R, Frieden IJ, et al. Timolol maleate 0.5% or 0.1% gel-forming solution for infantile hemangiomas: a retrospective, multicenter, cohort study. Pediatr Dermatol 2012;29(1): 28–31.

63. Chambers CB, Katowitz WR, Katowitz JA, et al. A controlled study of topical 0.25% timolol maleate gel for the treatment of cutaneous infantile capillary hemangiomas. Ophthal Plast Reconstr Surg 2012; 28(2):103–6.

64. Hynes S, Narasimhan K, Courtemanche DJ, et al. Complicated infantile hemangioma of the lip: outcomes of early versus late resection. Plast Reconstr Surg 2013;131(3):373e–9e.

65. Watanabe S, Takagi S, Sato Y, et al. Early surgical intervention for Japanese children with infantile hemangioma of the craniofacial region. J Craniofac Surg 2009;20(Suppl 1):707–9.

66. Lee AH, Hardy KL, Goltsman D, et al. A retrospective study to classify surgical indications for infantile hemangiomas. J Plast Reconstr Aesthet Surg 2014;67(9):1215–21.

67. Frieden IJ, Haggstrom AN, Drolet BA, et al. Infantile hemangiomas: current knowledge, future directions. Proceedings of a research workshop on infantile hemangiomas, April 7-9, 2005, Bethesda, Maryland, USA. Pediatr Dermatol 2005; 22(5):383–406.

68. Zide BM, Glat PM, Stile FL, et al. Vascular lip enlargement: part I. Hemangiomas–tenets of therapy. Plast Reconstr Surg 1997;100(7):1664–73.

69. Li WY, Chaudhry O, Reinisch JF. Guide to early surgical management of lip hemangiomas based on our experience of 214 cases. Plast Reconstr Surg 2011;128(5):1117–24.

70. Anderson RR, Parrish JA. Selective photothermolysis: precise microsurgery by selective absorption of pulsed radiation. Science 1983; 220(4596):524–7.

71. Kim HJ, Colombo M, Frieden IJ. Ulcerated hemangiomas: clinical characteristics and response to therapy. J Am Acad Dermatol 2001;44(6): 962–72.

72. Morelli JG, Tan OT, Weston WL. Treatment of ulcerated hemangiomas with the pulsed tunable dye laser. Am J Dis Child 1991;145(9):1062–4.

73. Wananukul S, Chatproedprai S. Ulcerated hemangiomas: clinical features and management. J Med Assoc Thai 2002;85(11):1220–5.

74. David LR, Malek MM, Argenta LC. Efficacy of pulse dye laser therapy for the treatment of ulcerated haemangiomas: a review of 78 patients. Br J Plast Surg 2003;56(4):317–27.

75. Witman PM, Wagner AM, Scherer K, et al. Complications following pulsed dye laser treatment of superficial hemangiomas. Lasers Surg Med 2006; 38(2):116–23.

76. Ashinoff R, Geronemus RG. Capillary hemangiomas and treatment with the flash lamp-pumped pulsed dye laser. Arch Dermatol 1991;127(2): 202–5.

77. Garden JM, Bakus AD, Paller AS. Treatment of cutaneous hemangiomas by the flashlamp-pumped pulsed dye laser: prospective analysis. J Pediatr 1992;120(4 Pt 1):555–60.

78. Landthaler M, Hohenleutner U, el-Raheem TA. Laser therapy of childhood haemangiomas. Br J Dermatol 1995;133(2):275–81.

79. Poetke M, Philipp C, Berlien HP. Flashlamp-pumped pulsed dye laser for hemangiomas in infancy: treatment of superficial vs mixed hemangiomas. Arch Dermatol 2000;136(5):628–32.

80. Kono T, Sakurai H, Groff WF, et al. Comparison study of a traditional pulsed dye laser versus a long-pulsed dye laser in the treatment of early childhood hemangiomas. Lasers Surg Med 2006; 38(2):112–5.

81. Rizzo C, Brightman L, Chapas AM, et al. Outcomes of childhood hemangiomas treated with the pulsed-dye laser with dynamic cooling: a retrospective chart analysis. Dermatol Surg 2009; 35(12):1947–54.

82. Hunzeker CM, Geronemus RG. Treatment of superficial infantile hemangiomas of the eyelid using the 595-nm pulsed dye laser. Dermatol Surg 2010; 36(5):590–7.

83. Hohenleutner S, Badur-Ganter E, Landthaler M, et al. Long-term results in the treatment of childhood hemangioma with the flashlamp-pumped pulsed dye laser: an evaluation of 617 cases. Lasers Surg Med 2001;28(3):273–7.

84. Batta K, Goodyear HM, Moss C, et al. Randomised controlled study of early pulsed dye laser treatment of uncomplicated childhood haemangiomas: results of a 1-year analysis. Lancet 2002;360(9332): 521–7.

85. Koay AC, Choo MM, Nathan AM, et al. Combined low-dose oral propranolol and oral prednisolone as first-line treatment in periocular infantile hemangiomas. J Ocul Pharmacol Ther 2011;27(3):309–11.

86. Reddy KK, Blei F, Brauer JA, et al. Retrospective study of the treatment of infantile hemangiomas using a combination of propranolol and pulsed dye laser. Dermatol Surg 2013;39(6):923–33.

87. Park KH, Jang YH, Chung HY, et al. Topical timolol maleate 0.5% for infantile hemangioma; it's effectiveness and/or adjunctive pulsed dye laser - single center experience of 102 cases in Korea. J Dermatolog Treat 2014;1–3. [Epub ahead of print].

88. Herschthal J, Wulkan A, George M, et al. Additive effect of propranolol and pulsed dye laser for infantile hemangioma. Dermatol Online J 2013;19(6): 18570.

89. Yuan KH, Li Q, Yu WL, et al. Successful combination therapy for severe infantile hemangiomas: case report and literature search. Photomed Laser Surg 2009;27(6):973–7.

90. Ehsani AH, Noormohammadpoor P, Abdolreza M, et al. Combination therapy of infantile hemangioma with pulsed dye laser with topical propranolol: a randomized clinical trial. Arch Iran Med 2014; 17(10):657–60.

91. Tamayo L, Ortiz DM, Orozco-Covarrubias L, et al. Therapeutic efficacy of interferon alfa-2b in infants with life-threatening giant hemangiomas. Arch Dermatol 1997;133(12):1567–71.

92. Ezekowitz RA, Mulliken JB, Folkman J. Interferon alfa-2a therapy for life-threatening hemangiomas of infancy. N Engl J Med 1992;326(22):1456–63.

93. Barlow CF, Priebe CJ, Mulliken JB, et al. Spastic diplegia as a complication of interferon alfa-2a treatment of hemangiomas of infancy. J Pediatr 1998;132(3 Pt 1):527–30.

94. Dubois J, Hershon L, Carmant L, et al. Toxicity profile of interferon alfa-2b in children: A prospective evaluation. J Pediatr 1999;135(6):782–5.

95. Michaud AP, Bauman NM, Burke DK, et al. Spastic diplegia and other motor disturbances in infants receiving interferon-alpha. Laryngoscope 2004; 114(7):1231–6.

96. Enjolras O, Brevière GM, Roger G, et al. Vincristine treatment for function- and life-threatening infantile hemangioma [in French]. Arch Pediatr 2004;11(2): 99–107.

97. Perez J, Pardo J, Gomez C. Vincristine–an effective treatment of corticoid-resistant life-threatening infantile hemangiomas. Acta Oncol 2002;41(2): 197–9.

98. Fawcett SL, Grant I, Hall PN, et al. Vincristine as a treatment for a large haemangioma threatening vital functions. Br J Plast Surg 2004;57(2):168–71.

99. Moore J, Lee M, Garzon M, et al. Effective therapy of a vascular tumor of infancy with vincristine. J Pediatr Surg 2001;36(8):1273–6.

100. Fukushima H, Kudo T, Fuskushima T, et al. An infant with life-threatening hemangioma successfully treated with low-dose cyclophosphamide. Pediatr Int 2011;53(6):1073–5.

101. Hurvitz SA, Hurvitz CH, Sloninsky L, et al. Successful treatment with cyclophosphamide of life-threatening diffuse hemangiomatosis involving the liver. J Pediatr Hematol Oncol 2000;22(6):527–32.

102. Gottschling S, Schneider G, Meyer S, et al. Two infants with life-threatening diffuse neonatal hemangiomatosis treated with cyclophosphamide. Pediatr Blood Cancer 2006;46(2):239–42.

103. Sovinz P, Urban C, Hausegger K. Life-threatening hemangiomatosis of the liver in an infant: multimodal therapy including cyclophosphamide and secondary acute myeloid leukemia. Pediatr Blood Cancer 2006;47(7):972–3.

104. Martinez MI, Sanchez-Carpintero I, North PE, et al. Infantile hemangioma: clinical resolution with 5% imiquimod cream. Arch Dermatol 2002;138(7): 881–4 [discussion: 884].

105. Qiu Y, Ma G, Yang J, et al. Imiquimod 5% cream versus timolol 0.5% ophthalmic solution for treating superficial proliferating infantile haemangiomas: a retrospective study. Clin Exp Dermatol 2013; 38(8):845–50.

106. Hazen PG, Carney JF, Engstrom CW, et al. Proliferating hemangioma of infancy: successful treatment with topical 5% imiquimod cream. Pediatr Dermatol 2005;22(3):254–6.

107. Jiang C, Hu X, Ma G, et al. A prospective self-controlled phase II study of imiquimod 5% cream in the treatment of infantile hemangioma. Pediatr Dermatol 2011;28(3):259–66.

108. Barry RB, Hughes BR, Cook LJ. Involution of infantile haemangiomas after imiquimod 5% cream. Clin Exp Dermatol 2008;33(4):446–9.

109. Burns AJ, Navarro JA. Role of laser therapy in pediatric patients. Plast Reconstr Surg 2009;124(1 Suppl):82e–92e.

110. Ulrich H, Bäumler W, Hohenleutner U, et al. Neodymium-YAG Laser for hemangiomas and vascular malformations – long term results. J Dtsch Dermatol Ges 2005;3(6):436–40.

111. Clymer MA, Fortune DS, Reinisch L, et al. Interstitial Nd:YAG photocoagulation for vascular malformations and hemangiomas in childhood. Arch Otolaryngol Head Neck Surg 1998;124(4):431–6.

Early Practice Focus
Evidence-Based Practice in Facial Plastic Surgery

James Teng, MD, J. Jared Christophel, MD, MPH*

KEYWORDS

- Evidence-based medicine • Level of evidence • Patient-reported outcome measures
- Observer-reported outcome measures

KEY POINTS

- Evidence-based medicine combines physician experience, knowledge of current literature, and patient preferences.
- Levels of evidence (LOE), determined by the design of the study, are applied to studies pertaining to clinical treatments and outcomes.
- The LOE should not imply a sense of quality, as there are studies with low LOE that provide strong recommendations, and likewise there are studies with high LOE that are flawed or fail to provide strong recommendations.
- Patient-reported outcome measures in facial plastic surgery evaluate quality of life, functional impact, disability, and body image.
- Expert data collection can be applied to facial nerve function, scar assessment, and facial rejuvenation.

INTRODUCTION/OVERVIEW OF EVIDENCE-BASED MEDICINE

The introduction of evidence-based medicine (EBM), defined by Sackett and colleagues[1] as "the conscientious, explicit, and judicious use of current best evidence in making decisions about the care of individual patients," caused a paradigm shift in how medicine is practiced. Medical schools and graduate medical education now incorporate EBM into training of medical students and residents. EBM, however, is a lifelong practice, and is thus important to continue even after graduation from residency. At its core, EBM incorporates 3 basic concepts: using the best research evidence available, applying the clinical expertise of the clinician, and understanding patient values.[1] It is important for the practicing facial plastic surgeon

to understand these concepts inherent in EBM so as to improve the health outcomes of patients and improve the quality of research in the field.

Incorporation of EBM into practice, more specifically, involves formulating clinically relevant questions, collecting the appropriate information, evaluating results, and applying the information to patient care. In this article, we aim to provide the building blocks to understanding and practicing EBM:

1. Understanding level of evidence and strength of recommendations in clinically relevant literature
2. Keeping updated with current literature and recommendations, and knowing where to search for pertinent information regarding specific clinical questions

Department of Otolaryngology - Head and Neck Surgery, University of Virginia Health System, PO Box 800713, Charlottesville, VA 22903, USA
* Corresponding author.
E-mail address: jjc3y@virginia.edu

Facial Plast Surg Clin N Am 23 (2015) 393–405
http://dx.doi.org/10.1016/j.fsc.2015.04.010
1064-7406/15/$ – see front matter © 2015 Elsevier Inc. All rights reserved.

3. Collection of data (patient-reported, observer-reported, and objective photodocumentation)
4. Evaluation of results and application to patient care as well as personal development

LEVELS OF EVIDENCE

Levels of evidence (LOE) are designations from the Oxford Centre for Evidence-Based Medicine (OCEBM) scale that stratify "likely best evidence" based on rigor of study design and susceptibility to bias. It was designed to act as a shortcut to assist clinicians in rapid appraisal of the available evidence; searching for studies based on LOE allows clinicians to efficiently narrow down searches to manageable quantities. LOE is assigned only to clinical and therapeutic studies. Studies that are basic science, non–human-based, diagnostic, and cadaver-based are not assigned LOE.[2] The hierarchy of evidence (**Table 1**) assigns LOE in ascending order starting with the expert opinion, assigned the lowest LOE score of 5, and ending with randomized controlled trials (RCTs) and meta-analyses, assigned the highest LOE score of 1. However, a higher LOE does not necessarily indicate more useful evidence, as studies with higher LOEs are typically associated with common diseases and more uncommon and rarer diseases are associated with lower LOEs.[3] Similarly, the surgical literature has been shown to have more studies associated with lower LOE, whereas studies dealing with nonsurgical treatment modalities tend to have higher LOE.[4]

Although LOE can provide insight into the quality of study design, it is important to understand that LOE does not evaluate the quality of evidence within a particular study. Similarly, LOE designation does not provide recommendations with any degree of certainty, as that decision must be made based on several factors: the clinician's background knowledge of the disease process and available treatment options, the similarities of study population characteristics to the patient, and the compatibility of patient values and circumstances with the treatment option.[2]

STRENGTH OF RECOMMENDATIONS

The strength of a clinical recommendation is equally important and complementary to knowledge of the LOE. It is important to understand the distinction between quality of evidence and strength of recommendation, as failure to distinguish the 2 may lead to confusion. A weak recommendation may be provided despite high quality of evidence; likewise, low quality of evidence can result in strong recommendations. Of the classification systems available, the GRADE (Grades of Recommendation, Assessment, Development, and Evaluation) approach assesses the quality of evidence and strength of recommendations in health care, and has been widely adopted by organizations including the World Health Organization, the American College of Physicians, and the Cochrane Collaboration.[5] This system is distinct from the LOE assigned by the OCEBM, and uses its own criteria to assess both quality of evidence and subsequent strength of recommendations (**Table 2**).[6] Quality of evidence is graded high, moderate, low, or very low. Strength of recommendations are strong or weak, and for or against using an intervention. Factors that affect the strength of recommendation include quality of evidence, uncertainty about the balance between desirable and undesirable effects, patient values and preferences, and whether the intervention represents a wise use of resources.

The American Academy of Pediatrics uses another classification scheme that has been adopted by several other resources.[7] This system evaluates both quality of evidence and strength of recommendations. Grades of evidence are similar to other classification schemes, with RCTs receiving the highest grades and observational studies receiving the lowest grades. Statements based on evidence are given strong recommendations, recommendations, option, or no recommendation.

Table 1
Levels of evidence from Oxford Centre For Evidence-Based Medicine

Level of Study	Types of Studies
Level 1	Randomized controlled trial (RCT) or meta-analysis of RCTs
Level 2	Prospective (cohort or outcomes) study with an internal control group or meta-analysis or prospective, controlled studies
Level 3	Retrospective (case-control) study with an internal control group or a meta-analysis of retrospective, controlled studies
Level 4	Case series without an internal control group, retrospective reviews, uncontrolled cohort studies
Level 5	Expert opinion without explicit critical appraisal, or on the basis of physiology/bench research

Adapted from OCEBM Levels of Evidence Working Group. "The Oxford levels of evidence 2." Oxford Centre for Evidence-Based Medicine. Available at: http://www.cebm.net/index.aspx?o=5653. Accessed April 16, 2015; with permission.

Table 2
Strength of recommendations from the GRADE system

Recommendation	Strength of Recommendation
1	Strong recommendation for using an intervention
2	Weak recommendation for using an intervention
3	Weak recommendation against using an intervention
4	Strong recommendation against using an intervention

Abbreviation: GRADE, Grades of Recommendation, Assessment, Development, and Evaluation.

Adapted from Guyatt GH, Oxman AD, Kunz R, et al. Going from evidence to recommendations. BMJ 2008;336(7652):1051; with permission.

Table 3
Resources available for evidence-based medicine

Type of Resource	Examples
Academic journals	*The Laryngoscope, Otolaryngology—Head and Neck Surgery, JAMA Facial Plastic Surgery*
Online databases	UpToDate, Cochrane Reviews, National Guidelines Clearinghouse, Essential Evidence Plus
E-mail updates	Daily POEMs ("Patient-Oriented Evidence that Matters") from Essential Evidence Plus

RESOURCES FOR EVIDENCE-BASED MEDICINE

Staying updated on current evidence can be challenging during practice. Fortunately, there are many resources for current evidence available in different forms of media. Major journal publications now assign LOE to articles regarding therapeutic and clinical topics. Committees and expert panels frequently publish guidelines that incorporate the most updated EBM, and provide recommendations with corresponding strengths of recommendations. Online reviews and databases, such as the Cochrane Review, are repositories of EBM. Online journal Web sites provide options for e-mail alerts to notify subscribers of new EBM articles. Additionally, subscribers can sign up for daily or weekly e-mails from these Web sites that highlight new and upcoming articles and provide synopses. A summary of various resources for EBM are compiled in **Table 3**.

INCORPORATING EVIDENCE-BASED MEDICINE INTO PRACTICE

Practicing EBM is more than just staying current on the best clinical evidence; it involves incorporating the guidelines in clinical decision-making and collecting outcome measure data on patients. Incorporating guidelines in clinical decision-making often requires an algorithmic approach, and can be implemented with the help of the electronic medical record. Collecting outcome data allows for more precise, reliable data points with

which to make the clinical decisions, as well as give the surgeon feedback about how he or she is performing.

OUTCOME MEASURES

Outcome measures are becoming increasingly prevalent in EBM. They can be classified as patient-reported outcomes measures (PROMs) or clinical or efficacy outcomes (expert data collection). Patient-reported outcomes primarily involve questionnaires assessing quality of life (QOL) or patient satisfaction regarding a health-related condition. Clinical outcomes, on the other hand, involve objective and observational assessments, and are used in case-control studies, cohort studies, and RCTs.[8]

On a larger scale, outcome measures are driving health care funding and reimbursement at the governmental level. The Agency for Health Care Research and Quality uses outcome measures to make recommendations to other Department of Health and Human Services agencies like the Centers for Medicare and Medicaid Services. Two of the most common outcome measures used to assess global individual function are the Short Form-36 and activities of daily living. When creating other outcome measures (such as those specific to facial plastic surgery), these often serve as the referent standard with which to compare reliability and consistency. Surgeries performed by facial plastic and reconstructive surgeons (FPRSs) will eventually come under more rigorous outcome measure scrutiny and will have to prove effective. Although few FPRS-specific patient-reported and clinical outcome measures existed decades ago, more outcome measures have been created over the past few decades and have been validated in multiple studies.

Most FPRS outcome measures have focused on clinical outcomes, but patient QOL and functional outcomes are trending and are being incorporated into outcome measures. The scope of outcome measures in facial plastic surgery encompasses a multitude of patient-reported scales and observer-reported scales, including facial nerve grading systems, scar-assessment scales, and facial wrinkle scales.[8] Here we review several of the more commonly used outcome measures used in facial plastic surgery.

EXPERT DATA COLLECTION
Facial Nerve Grading Systems

Facial nerve assessment is one of the most commonly studied outcome measures in both facial plastic surgery and otolaryngology. Grading facial nerve injury is necessary to communicate and document severity of injury and improvement of function with treatment. Several objective grading scales of facial nerve injury have been created and are regularly used. These scales focus on the appearance of resting symmetry and symmetry during voluntary motion. Synkinesis, abnormal involuntary facial movement that occurs with voluntary movement of different facial muscle groups due to abnormal regeneration of facial nerve fibers, has been incorporated into more recently created facial nerve grading scales.

The House-Brackmann Facial Nerve Grading System (HBFNGS), first introduced in 1983 and then adopted by the Facial Nerve Disorders Committee of the American Academy of Otolaryngology—Head and Neck Surgery in 1984, has been validated in numerous studies and has been widely used in multiple clinical applications.[9] This system evaluates facial asymmetry at rest and in motion. Gross observations are made in comparison with the normal side. Facial motion is evaluated based on facial thirds (upper third: forehead, middle third: eye, lower third: mouth). The grading system determines severity of injury, from normal (House-Brackmann Grade I) to total paralysis (House-Brackmann Grade VI), based on degree of movement and gross asymmetry as determined by the observer (**Table 4**). Despite its widespread use and applicability, there are limitations to the grading system. The application of a single grade represents the global function of the facial nerve, but there actually may be varying levels of functional impairment to different facial muscle groups. Although typically the grade reflects the poorest functioning muscle group, other more functional muscle groups may not be adequately

Table 4 House-Brackmann facial nerve grading system	
Grade	**Description**
I	Normal function, no asymmetry
II	Mild dysfunction, slight weakness, complete eye closure, barely perceptible asymmetry
III	Moderate dysfunction, complete eye closure, asymmetry with motion
IV	Moderately severe dysfunction, incomplete eye closure, obvious asymmetry with motion, normal symmetry at rest
V	Severe dysfunction, barely perceptible motion with maximal effort, asymmetry at rest
VI	Total paralysis, no movement, obvious asymmetry

characterized with a single grade. A study by Reitzen and colleagues[9] in 2009 showed that a single grade did not fully communicate facial function, but that regional assessment of different facial muscle groups more accurately communicated facial function.

The Sunnybrook Facial Grading System (SFGS) was introduced by Ross and colleagues in 1992.[10] Resting symmetry, symmetry of voluntary movement, and synkinesis are separately scored and a composite score is totaled from the sum of the 3 individual categories (**Fig. 1**). Numerical values are assigned based on degree of asymmetry or movement; higher composite scores indicate more normal function, whereas lower composite scores correlate with poorer function. Resting asymmetry is evaluated at the eye, nasolabial fold, and mouth. Voluntary movement is evaluated by using separate facial motions involving distinct facial muscle groups: brow lift (frontalis), eye closure (orbicularis oculi), open mouth smile (zygomaticus major, risorius), snarl (levator labii superioris, levator labii superior alaeque nasi), and lip pucker (orbicularis oris). Synkinesis is simultaneously assessed when evaluating the previously mentioned facial muscle groups. Compared with the HBFNGS, which focuses more on global assessment, the SFGS is a more regionally weighted system. The 2 systems are widely used, and conversion tables have been created to translate HBFNGS grades to SFGS scores and vice versa.[11] Validation studies have concluded that the SFGS is the most objective of the current facial nerve grading systems, with comparable repeatability and improved interrater agreement compared with the HBFNGS.[12]

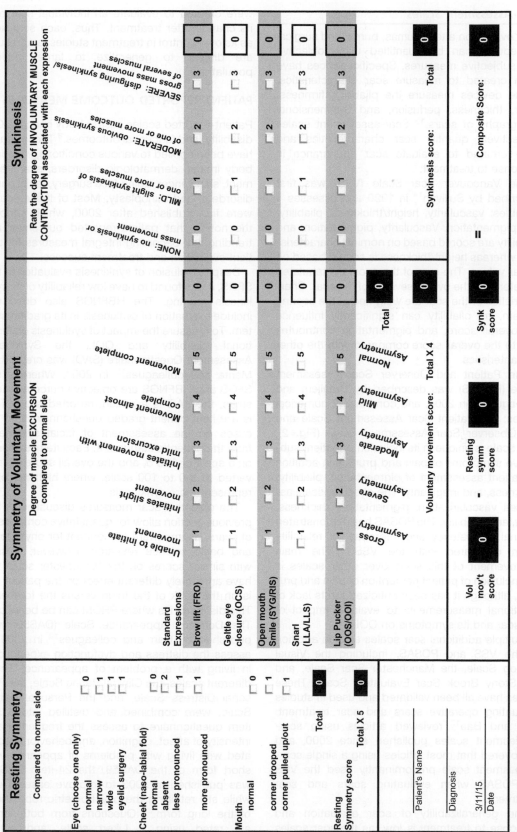

Fig. 1. Sunnybrook facial grading system. (Available at: http://sunnybrook.ca/uploads/FacialGradingSystem.pdf. Accessed April 16, 2015; with permission.)

Scar-Assessment Scales

Scar evaluation after traumas, burns, and surgical procedures can be quantified using objective and subjective measures. Specific devices have been created to measure scar characteristics. These devices measure the pliability, firmness, color, thickness, perfusion, and 3-dimensional topography of scars.[13] Scar-assessment scales subjectively quantify scar characteristics and were created to evaluate scar appearance in response to treatment.

The Vancouver Scar Scale (VSS) was first described by Sullivan[14] in 1990 and assesses 4 variables: vascularity, height/thickness, pliability, and pigmentation. Vascularity, pigmentation, and pliability are scored based on nominal characteristics, whereas height/thickness is scored based on scalar values. The sum of the scores is tabulated to determine the overall severity of the scar. Characteristics of the scar are weighted in the scoring system, as pliability can significantly influence the overall score, and pigmentation contributes less to the overall score compared with the other characteristics.

The Patient and Observer Scar Assessment Scale (POSAS) was described by Draaijers and colleagues[15] in 2004, and combines 2 numerical scales: the Patient Scar Assessment Scale and the Observer Scar Assessment Scale (**Fig. 2**). This scale is unique in its inclusion of patient subjective symptoms of pain and pruritus in addition to patient assessment of pigmentation, pliability, thickness, and irregularity. The observer scale assesses vascularization, pigmentation, thickness, relief, and pliability. The POSAS has demonstrated internal consistency and interobserver reliability when compared with the VSS.[16] The main improvement of this scale over other scales is the inclusion of patient perception of pain and pruritus, although it has been criticized for its lack of functional measurements to evaluate impact of the scar and its symptoms on QOL.[16]

Multiple additional scar scales exist in addition to the VSS and POSAS, including the Visual Analog Scale, the Manchester Scar Scale, and the Stony Brook Scar Evaluation Scale. These scales have all been validated and used in studies evaluating operative scars and scar treatment. Bae and Bae[17] reviewed articles using scar-assessment scales published since 2000, and discovered that most articles using a single scar-assessment scale predominantly used the VSS or POSAS when evaluating scars and scar treatment.

The generalizability of scar evaluation and response to treatment is low, as the scar scales were created to evaluate an individual scar and its change after treatment. Thus, each scar acts as its own control in treatment studies, and results are difficult to generalize to larger patient populations.

PATIENT-REPORTED OUTCOME MEASURES

Patient-reported scales assess body image, QOL, disability, and functional outcomes.[8] These scales have been applied to various conditions, including body image, dermatologic disorders, scar treatment, skin cancer, aging face surgery, facial nerve disorders, and rhinoplasty. Most of these scales were first published after 2000, which support the notion that patient-reported outcomes are trending and becoming integral measures for patient evaluation and treatment success.

Despite inclusion of synkinesis evaluation in the SFGS, it was found to have low reliability of its synkinesis grading. The HBFNGS also does not include evaluation of synkinesis in its grading system. To measure the impact of synkinesis on functional disability and QOL, the Synkinesis Assessment Questionnaire (SAQ) was created by Mehta and colleagues[18] in 2007. Whereas the SFGS and HBFNGS are objective outcome measures, the SAQ is a patient-reported scale. This is a 9-item patient-graded questionnaire that focuses on the assessment of facial synkinesis from the patient's standpoint. Each item is scored on a scale of 1 to 5, and the overall score is converted to a 0 to 100 scale, where higher scores represent more synkinesis.[18]

The objective scar measures discussed in the previous section allow for quantitative comparison of scars, an important component for physiologic and basic science research. However, a scar with similar scores on the Manchester scale will have an entirely different effect on the patient if it is on the back of the thigh versus the forehead. This distinction is where PROM can be beneficial. The Derriford Appearance Scale (DAS59) was published by Carr and colleagues[19] in 2000 to assess the distress and dysfunction experienced in living with a problem of appearance. Three different scales, the Clinical Rating Scale, the Personal Distress Scale, and the Personal Rating Scale, were combined and distilled into a 59-item questionnaire to assess the frequency and intensity of affect, cognition, and behavior associated with living with problems of appearance. A short form of the DAS59, the 24-item DAS24, was published in 2005 to improve ease of use while still retaining the psychometric robustness of the long form.[20] Questions from both forms are rated using a Likert scale, and higher

POSAS Patient scale

A

The Patient and Observer Scar Assessment Scale v2.0 / EN

Date of examination: _____

Observer: _____

Location: _____

Research / study: _____

Name of patient: _____

Date of birth: _____

Identification number: _____

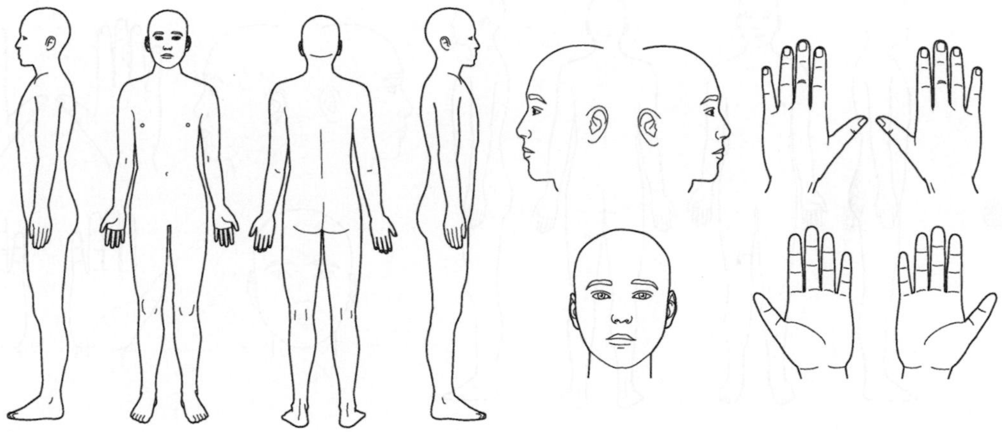

1 = no, not at all   **yes, very much = 10**

① ② ③ ④ ⑤ ⑥ ⑦ ⑧ ⑨ ⑩

HAS THE SCAR BEEN PAINFUL THE PAST FEW WEEKS?

HAS THE SCAR BEEN ITCHING THE PAST FEW WEEKS?

1 = no, as normal skin   **yes, very different = 10**

IS THE SCAR COLOR DIFFERENT FROM THE COLOR OF YOUR NORMAL SKIN AT PRESENT?

IS THE STIFFNESS OF THE SCAR DIFFERENT FROM YOUR NORMAL SKIN AT PRESENT?

IS THE THICKNESS OF THE SCAR DIFFERENT FROM YOUR NORMAL SKIN AT PRESENT?

IS THE SCAR MORE IRREGULAR THAN YOUR NORMAL SKIN AT PRESENT?

1 = as normal skin   **very different = 10**

① ② ③ ④ ⑤ ⑥ ⑦ ⑧ ⑨ ⑩

WHAT IS YOUR OVERALL OPINION OF THE SCAR COMPARED TO NORMAL SKIN?

Fig. 2. POSAS. The POSAS consists of 2 different scales: the (*A*) patient scale and the (*B*) observer scale. (Available at: http://www.posas.org/downloads/english. Accessed April 16, 2015; with permission.)

cumulative scores indicate increasing levels of distress and dysfunction associated with body image. Both forms have been validated in multiple studies, and in addition to general body image,

can be applied to esthetic surgery, facial trauma, scarring, and facial paralysis.[8]

The Nasal Obstruction Symptom Evaluation (NOSE) scale, first published by Stewart and

B POSAS Observer scale

The Patient and Observer Scar Assessment Scale v2.0 / EN

Date of examination: _____

Observer: _____

Location: _____

Research / study: _____

Name of patient: _____

Date of birth: _____

Identification number: _____

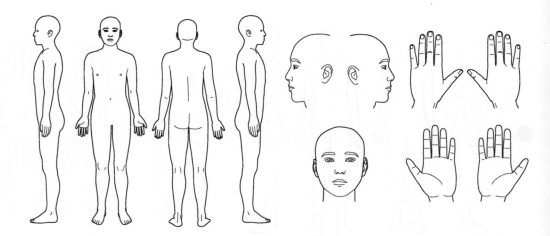

Explanation

The observer scale of the POSAS consists of six items (vascularity, pigmentation, thickness, relief, pliability and surface area).
All items are scored on a scale ranging from 1 ('like normal skin') to 10 ('worst scar imaginable').
The sum of the six items results in a total score of the POSAS observer scale. Categories boxes are added for each item. Furthermore, an overall opinion is scored on a scale ranging from 1 to 10.
All parameters should preferably be compared to normal skin on a comparable anatomic location.

Explanatory notes on the items:

- **VASCULARITY** Presence of vessels in scar tissue assessed by the amount of redness, tested by the amount of blood return after blanching with a piece of Plexiglas
- **PIGMENTATION** Brownish coloration of the scar by pigment (melanin); apply Plexiglas to the skin with moderate pressure to eliminate the effect of vascularity
- **THICKNESS** Average distance between the subcutical-dermal border and the epidermal surface of the scar
- **RELIEF** The extent to which surface irregularities are present (preferably compared with adjacent normal skin)
- **PLIABILITY** Suppleness of the scar tested by wrinkling the scar between the thumb and index finger
- **SURFACE AREA** Surface area of the scar in relation to the original wound area

Fig. 2. (continued)

colleagues[21] in 2004, is a 5-item questionnaire to assess subjective improvement in nasal obstruction treatment. The patient is asked to rate the severity of nasal congestion/stuffiness, nasal blockage/obstruction, difficulty with nasal airflow, sleep difficulty, and nasal breathing during exercise on a 5-point Likert scale (**Fig. 3**). The raw score ranges from 0 to 20, but is multiplied by 5

Nasal Obstruction and Septoplasty Effectiveness Scale

Physician AAO-HNS#:_____ Patient ID: _____ Today's date: __ /__ /__ __ __ __

→ **To the Patient:** Please help us to better understand the impact of nasal obstruction on your quality of life by **completing following survey**. Thank You!

Over the past _ONE_ month, how much of a problem were the following conditions for you?

Please ⟨circle⟩ the most correct response

	Not a Problem	_Very Mild Problem_	_Moderate problem_	_Fairly Bad Problem_	_Severe problem_
1. Nasal congestion or stuffiness	0	1	2	3	4
2. Nasal blockage or obstruction	0	1	2	3	4
3. Trouble breathing through my nose	0	1	2	3	4
4. Trouble sleeping	0	1	2	3	4
5. Unable to get enough air through my nose during exercise or exertion	0	1	2	3	4

Nasal Obstruction Symptom Evaluation Scale
©AAO-HNS Foundation 2002

Fig. 3. NOSE scale. (*Adapted from* Stewart MG, Witsell DL, Smith TL, et al. Development and validation of the nasal obstruction symptom evaluation (NOSE) scale. Otolaryngol Head Neck Surg 2004;130:162; with permission.)

to scale the final score from 0 to 100, so a score of 0 indicates no problems with nasal obstruction and a score of 100 indicates the most severe problems. The NOSE scale has been used to assess disease-specific QOL outcomes after nasal septoplasty in patients with nasal obstruction.[22] This scale has been evaluated in multiple studies, has been translated into multiple different languages, and has been shown to be both reliable and validated.[8,23,24]

Aging Face and Facial Rejuvenation Assessment Scales

The success of esthetic facial plastic surgery and facial rejuvenation procedures is dependent on the surgeon's or observer's satisfaction with the results of surgery, but also the patient's perception of the results of surgery. It can be argued that the patient's satisfaction is by far the most important indicator of successful surgery. Each patient's assessment of results is influenced by individual character and personality traits. The purpose of PROMs in esthetic surgery is to standardize assessment of these results, making them useful in research.

The Rhinoplasty Outcomes Evaluation, Facelift Outcomes Evaluation, Blepharoplasty Outcomes Evaluation, and Skin Rejuvenation Outcomes Evaluation were introduced by Alsarraf[25] in 2000. Each instrument consists of 6 items and evaluates outcomes relating to physical, mental, and social functioning after a procedure. Each instrument is customized in response to the procedure performed, and in addition assesses the desire for revision. Each item is scored from 0 to 4, and the cumulative score is converted to a 0 to 100 scale, with 0 indicating the least patient satisfaction and

100 indicating the most satisfaction. Each instrument was constructed using expert opinion, and has tested well for reliability and validity.[26]

The Facial Line Treatment Satisfaction Questionnaire has 14 items that assess patient satisfaction with facial line treatment using botulinum toxin type A.[27] This was created by industry professionals in 2003. The items in the questionnaire assess satisfaction with both treatment effects and the procedure. Pilot testing was conducted on patients undergoing esthetic treatment for facial lines, and has been validated.

Many PROMs used in esthetic facial surgery underwent limited development and validation before publication.[28] Several instruments reviewed by Kosowski and colleagues were developed using expert opinion alone. Overall, their review concluded that valid, reliable, and responsive instruments in esthetic facial surgery were lacking.[28]

Data storage, research preparedness, and the Health Insurance Portability and Accountability Act

Collecting and analyzing data involves obtaining institutional review board (IRB) approval, obtaining patient consent for data and photo collection, storing information and photodocumentation, and assessment of outcome measures.

As discussed, collecting outcome measures is an important part of EBM. In the past, most researchers have collected outcome measures prospectively separate from the electronic medical record (EMR) in IRB-approved databases. With the advent of newer EMRs, the outcome measures can be incorporated into the visit note with smart phrases and drop down menus and become part of the EMR. This later method has the advantages of increasing medicolegal documentation, does not require IRB approval to collect (it is part of the EMR), and is often simpler to implement. To perform research on outcome measures collected this way, IRB approval still must be obtained to do retrospective collection. The benefit of the prospective database method is that the important data points for the study already have been extracted.

Photographs and videos are important data points for facial plastic surgeons. Consent for photodocumentation must be obtained before any photography. Patient consent should understand that photographs are part of the medical record for medicolegal documentation, and also may be used for educations purposes, including lectures, posters, and publications.

Photodocumentation should be standardized for specific surgical procedures. Rhinoplasty, mentoplasty, otoplasty, blepharoplasty,

rhytidectomy/facial animation, browplasty, lip augmentation, and cleft lip repair each use specific photographic series that use specific views. Henderson and colleagues[29] article on photographic standards in facial plastic surgery provides an overview of procedures and associated views. Patient positioning should be along the Frankfurt horizontal line. Deviation from this with neck flexion/extension and head protrusion/retrusion can alter the appearance of the submental area, jawline, and melolabial groove.[30] Hair should be put up to expose the face and brow. Jewelry, eyeglasses, and other distractors should be removed. Makeup should be removed when documenting skin conditions before skin resurfacing procedures.[29]

Protected health information (PHI) should be stored on secured storage devices and servers. Portable data storage devices, such as Universal Serial Bus (USB) drives or external hard drives, should incorporate encryption and password protection before allowing the user to store or access PHI. Encryption of storage devices can be either hardware-based or software-based.[31] Hardware-based encryption uses a dedicated processor physically located on the encrypted device, is "always on," and does not require driver or software installation on the host computer. Multiple manufacturers have made these devices available for the purpose of transporting secure data, primarily in the corporate setting. Software-based encryption requires computer resources to encrypt data, requires periodic software updates, and is only as secure as the host computer. Encryption software is readily available, can be used with any storage device, and is cost-effective in smaller settings.

Internet data storage services, commonly referred to as "the cloud," are becoming more popular for data backup and storage of large files. Cloud storage has the added benefit of accessibility across a wide range of devices, including computers, tablets, and mobile devices. Commercially available cloud-storage services are generally reliable and use techniques such as password-authentication, encryption, and authorization practices for security. However, these security practices do not guarantee invulnerability from attempts at data theft from hackers, which is a common concern of cloud-storage users. In addition, to store PHI on any third-party service (eg, box, Dropbox, Amazon, iCloud), the user would need a business associate agreement (BAA) with the service. The BAA is specific to HIPAA (Health Insurance Portability and Accountability Act) and ensures the third party is responsible for encryption and protection of the data. The BAA is typically already in place for clinical trial repositories or dedicated case logs in the cloud (eg, REDCap, American College of Surgeons Case Log), but almost nonexistent for other mainstream services already mentioned. Network-attached storage uses a hard drive with network connectivity to allow access to devices within a designated network. Access to the network should be through a firewall, which prohibits unauthorized users from accessing information on the storage device. For more information on how to securely store and access information, we recommend consulting an information technology specialist.

BARRIERS TO EVIDENCE-BASED MEDICINE

Despite widely available resources to access EBM publications and numerous scales to use for the basis of data collection, there are barriers to implementing EBM in daily practice. The initial introduction of EBM was met with concerns that EBM was a form of "cookbook" medicine based on algorithms and a threat to physician autonomy and individualized treatment decisions.[4] However, as noted by Sackett and colleagues,[1] EBM actually incorporates individual clinical expertise with understanding of the best available evidence and patient preference. EBM principles have been incorporated into medical school education now as the first step to establish a lifelong commitment to evidence-based practice. Graduate medical education, too, has begun to foster evidence-based practice in residents and fellows, although the negative influence of faculty members and their resistance to EBM can be a barrier to EBM.[32] Fortunately, program directors and resident educators have fostered evidence-based practice during training, thus establishing the foundations of EBM for a new generation of physicians.

Although a paradigm shift largely in support of EBM has taken place, there are still challenges to implementing EBM in the surgical literature. A review of articles making clinical recommendations published in otolaryngology journals showed that the LOE was significantly higher in studies making medical treatment recommendations versus surgical treatment recommendations.[4] Articles making medical and surgical treatment recommendations had LOE ranging from 1 to 4, but the overwhelming majority of studies making surgical treatment recommendations used uncontrolled studies (LOE 4) (86% vs 58%). Although there is a focus on developing and publishing studies with higher LOE, it is important for those reading and evaluating studies to understand the difference between LOE and quality. The LOE should not imply a sense of quality, as there are studies with low LOE that provide strong recommendations, and likewise there are studies with high LOE that are flawed or fail to provide strong recommendations.[32]

Isenberg and Rosenfield[33] outlined 5 major problems affecting otolaryngologists from participating in community-based outcomes research: overly long and complex surveys, lack of time during office hours, cumbersome data collection requirements, inadequate communication between principal investigator and participating physicians, and lack of enthusiasm. Many instruments reviewed in this article fortunately have few items to complete; longer and more detailed instruments, such as the DAS59, have been shortened to the DAS24 to be more easily used for research.

Ultimately, data gathered and analyzed for use in EBM should be applicable to daily practice. A new generation of technology allows integration of the electronic health record (EHR) and treatment recommendations based on current EBM. These technologies, known as Computerized Decision Support Systems (CDSSs), have been designed to aid clinical decision-making by using patient data referenced in the EHR.[34] Ideally, integration of these technologies into current practice should aid in patient care, decrease health care–associated costs, and decrease morbidity and mortality. Unfortunately, reviews of this burgeoning technology have not provided any evidence of improvement in mortality when using CDSSs, and only weak evidence for improving morbidity.[34] As more care is transitioned to the EHR, incorporation of CDSSs to clinical decision-making may take place, allowing more opportunity to study the effect of EBM on improving all aspects of health care.

SUMMARY

The importance of EBM cannot be stressed enough. As medicine becomes more outcome-oriented, outcome measures will be one of the rulers by which treatment utility and success is measured. Physicians and the treatments used will be increasingly scrutinized by both payers and patients, and will need to use outcome measures to grade their success and defend their uses. Here we provided an outline to what is involved in understanding EBM and incorporating it into daily practice. The degree of incorporation is variable depending on the practice setting, but the new paradigm for practicing medicine requires all physicians to pursue lifelong learning and improvement in practice.

REFERENCES

1. Sackett DL, Rosenberg WM, Gray JA, et al. Evidence based medicine: what it is and what it isn't. BMJ 1996;312(7023):71–2.

2. Howick J, Chalmers I, Glasziou P, et al. The 2011 oxford CEBM levels of evidence (introductory document). OCEBM Levels of Evidence Web site. 2011. Available at: http://www.cebm.net/wp-content/uploads/2014/06/CEBM-Levels-of-Evidence-Introduction-2.1.pdf. Accessed January 26, 2015.

3. Rhee JS, Daramola OO. No need to fear evidence-based medicine. Arch Facial Plast Surg 2012; 14(2):89–92.

4. Bentsianov BL, Boruk M, Rosenfeld RM. Evidence-based medicine in otolaryngology journals. Otolaryngol Head Neck Surg 2002;126(4):371–6.

5. Guyatt GH, Oxman AD, Vist GE, et al. GRADE: an emerging consensus on rating quality of evidence and strength of recommendations. BMJ 2008; 336(7650):924–6.

6. Guyatt GH, Oxman AD, Kunz R, et al. Going from evidence to recommendations. BMJ 2008; 336(7652):1049–51.

7. Homer C, Lannon C, Harbaugh N, et al. Classifying recommendations for clinical practice guidelines. Pediatrics 2004;114(3):874–7.

8. Rhee JS, McMullin BT. Outcome measures in facial plastic surgery: patient-reported and clinical efficacy measures. Arch Facial Plast Surg 2008;10(3):194–207.

9. Reitzen SD, Babb JS, Lalwani AK. Significance and reliability of the house-brackmann grading system for regional facial nerve function. Otolaryngol Head Neck Surg 2009;140(2):154–8.

10. Ross BG, Fradet G, Nedzelski JM. Development of a sensitive clinical facial grading system. Otolaryngol Head Neck Surg 1996;114(3):380–6.

11. Kanerva M, Jonsson L, Berg T, et al. Sunnybrook and house-brackmann systems in 5397 facial gradings. Otolaryngol Head Neck Surg 2011;144(4):570–4.

12. Kanerva M, Poussa T, Pitkäranta A. Sunnybrook and house-brackmann facial grading systems: intrarater repeatability and interrater agreement. Otolaryngol Head Neck Surg 2006;135(6):865–71.

13. Fearmonti R, Bond J, Erdmann D, et al. A review of scar scales and scar measuring devices. Eplasty 2010;10:e43.

14. Sullivan TA, Smith J, Kermode J, et al. Rating the burn scar. J Burn Care Res 1990;11(3):256–60.

15. Draaijers LJ, Tempelman FR, Botman YA, et al. The patient and observer scar assessment scale: a reliable and feasible tool for scar evaluation. Plast Reconstr Surg 2004;113(7):1960–5.

16. van de Kar AL, Corion LU, Smeulders MJ, et al. Reliable and feasible evaluation of linear scars by the patient and observer scar assessment scale. Plast Reconstr Surg 2005;116(2):514–22.

17. Bae SH, Bae YC. Analysis of frequency of use of different scar assessment scales based on the scar condition and treatment method. Arch Plast Surg 2014;41(2):111–5.

18. Mehta RP, WernickRobinson M, Hadlock TA. Validation of the synkinesis assessment questionnaire. Laryngoscope 2007;117(5):923–6.

19. Carr T, Harris D, James C. The derriford appearance scale (DAS-59): a new scale to measure individual responses to living with problems of appearance. Br J Health Psychol 2000;5(2):201–15.

20. Carr T, Moss T, Harris D. The DAS24: a short form of the derriford appearance scale DAS59 to measure individual responses to living with problems of appearance. Br J Health Psychol 2005;10(2): 285–98.

21. Stewart MG, Witsell DL, Smith TL, et al. Development and validation of the nasal obstruction symptom evaluation (NOSE) scale. Otolaryngol Head Neck Surg 2004;130(2):157–63.

22. Stewart MG, Smith TL, Weaver EM, et al. Outcomes after nasal septoplasty: results from the nasal obstruction septoplasty effectiveness (NOSE) study. Otolaryngol Head Neck Surg 2004;130(3):283–90.

23. Lachanas VA, Tsiouvaka S, Tsea M, et al. Validation of the nasal obstruction symptom evaluation (NOSE) scale for greek patients. Otolaryngol Head Neck Surg 2014;151(5):819–23.

24. Marro M, Mondina M, Stoll D, et al. French validation of the NOSE and RhinoQOL questionnaires in the management of nasal obstruction. Otolaryngol Head Neck Surg 2011;144(6):988–93.

25. Alsarraf R. Outcomes research in facial plastic surgery: a review and new directions. Aesthetic Plast Surg 2000;24(3):192–7.

26. Alsarraf R, Larrabee WF, Anderson S, et al. Measuring cosmetic facial plastic surgery outcomes: a pilot study. Arch Facial Plast Surg 2001; 3(3):198–201.

27. Cox SE, Finn JC, Stetler L, et al. Development of the facial lines treatment satisfaction questionnaire and initial results for botulinum toxin type A–Treated patients. Dermatol Surg 2003;29(5):444–9.

28. Kosowski TR, McCarthy C, Reavey PL, et al. A systematic review of patient-reported outcome measures after facial cosmetic surgery and/or nonsurgical facial rejuvenation. Plast Reconstr Surg 2009;123(6):1819–27.

29. Henderson JL, Larrabee WF, Krieger BD. Photographic standards for facial plastic surgery. Arch Facial Plast Surg 2005;7(5):331–3.

30. Sommer DD, Mendelsohn M. Pitfalls of nonstandardized photography in facial plastic surgery patients. Plast Reconstr Surg 2004;114(1):10–4.

31. Hardware- vs software-based encryption. Secure USB Flash Drives Web site. Available at: http://www.kingston.com/us/usb/encrypted_security/hardware_vs_software. Accessed January 26, 2015.

32. Eaves FF, Rohrich RJ, Sykes JM. Taking evidence-based plastic surgery to the next level: report of

the second summit on evidence-based plastic surgery. JAMA Facial Plast Surg 2013;15(4):314–20.

33. Isenberg SF, Rosenfeld RM. Problems and pitfalls in community-based outcomes research. Otolaryngol Head Neck Surg 1997;116(6 Pt 1):662–5.

34. Moja L, Kwag KH, Lytras T, et al. Effectiveness of computerized decision support systems linked to electronic health records: a systematic review and meta-analysis. Am J Public Health 2014;104(12): e12–22.

Index

Note: Page numbers of article titles are in **boldface** type.

Facial Plast Surg Clin N Am 23 (2015) 407–416

http://dx.doi.org/10.1016/S1064-7406(15)00062-0

Moving?

Make sure your subscription moves with you!

To notify us of your new address, find your Clinics Account Number (located on your mailing label above your name), and contact customer service at:

Email: journalscustomerservice-usa@elsevier.com

800-654-2452 (subscribers in the U.S. & Canada)
314-447-8871 (subscribers outside of the U.S. & Canada)

Fax number: 314-447-8029

Elsevier Health Sciences Division
Subscription Customer Service
3251 Riverport Lane
Maryland Heights, MO 63043

To ensure uninterrupted delivery of your subscription, please notify us at least 4 weeks in advance of move.

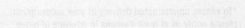

Printed and bound by CPI Group (UK) Ltd, Croydon, CR0 4YY

06/02/2024

01043712-0014

Printed and bound by CPI Group (UK) Ltd, Croydon, CR0 4YY
03/10/2024
01040378-0014